Quick Questions in the
Shoulder
Expert Advice in Sports Medicine

Quick Questions in Sports Medicine

Series

Series Editor, Eric L. Sauers, PhD, ATC, FNATA

Quick Questions in the Shoulder

Expert Advice in Sports Medicine

Editor

Kellie C. Huxel Bliven, PhD, ATC
Associate Professor, Kinesiology Program
College of Graduate Health Studies
A.T. Still University
Mesa, Arizona

Series Editor

Eric L. Sauers, PhD, ATC, FNATA
Professor and Chair
Department of Interdisciplinary Health Sciences
Arizona School of Health Sciences
A.T. Still University
Mesa, Arizona

Routledge
Taylor & Francis Group
NEW YORK AND LONDON

First published in 2015 by SLACK Incorporated

Published 2024 by Routledge
605 Third Avenue, New York, NY 10017
4 Park Square, Milton Park, Abingdon, Oxon OX14 4RN

Routledge is an imprint of the Taylor & Francis Group, an informa business

Library of Congress Cataloging-in-Publication Data
Quick questions in the shoulder : expert advice in sports medicine / editor, Kelly C. Huxel Bliven.
p. ; cm. -- (Quick questions in athletic training)
Includes bibliographical references and index.
ISBN 9781617119842 (paperback : alk. paper)
I. Bliven, Kelly C. Huxel, editor. II. National Athletic Trainers' Association, issuing body. III. Series: Quick questions in athletic training.
[DNLM: 1. Shoulder--injuries--Examination Questions. 2. Athletic Injuries--Examination Questions. WE 18.2]
RC1210
617.1'027076--dc23
2015008482

ISBN: 9781617119842 (pbk)
ISBN: 9781003526148 (ebk)

DOI: 10.4324/9781003526148

Dedication

To my family, especially my parents, Jim and Linda Huxel, and my husband, Chris. Thank you for your unending love, support, and encouragement through all of my pursuits. And to all of my teachers, mentors, colleagues, and students who positively influence and challenge me daily.

Contents

Acknowledgments

I would like to express my sincere appreciation to all of the contributing authors for their willingness to share their expertise for this project; thanks to Josie Harding for her assistance; and a special thank you to my friend and colleague, Gail Parr, for her editorial support throughout the project.

About the Editor

Kellie C. Huxel Bliven, PhD, ATC is an Associate Professor in the Kinesiology Program within the College of Graduate Health Studies at A.T. Still University (ATSU) in Mesa, Arizona. She is also an adjunct faculty member in anatomy for several residential programs at ATSU. Dr. Huxel Bliven earned her BA in biology and physical education from Denison University in Granville, Ohio; her MS in kinesiology from Indiana University in Bloomington, Indiana; and her PhD in kinesiology with an athletic training emphasis from Temple University in Philadelphia, Pennsylvania. Dr. Huxel Bliven has an active research line in the area of dynamic restraint of the shoulder, examining shoulder adaptations in overhead athletes, upper extremity muscle activation during rehabilitation exercises, and health-related quality of life in throwing athletes. Dr. Huxel Bliven serves on the Board of Certification's Exam Development Committee, is the Associate Editor for the *Journal of Sport Rehabilitation*, and is an active member in the American Society for Shoulder and Elbow Therapists (ASSET).

Contributing Authors

Barton E. Anderson, MS, AT, ATC (Questions 23, 38)
Assistant Professor and Clinical Education Coordinator, Athletic Training Programs
A.T. Still University
Mesa, Arizona

Amanda Arnold, PT, DPT, OCS, SCS (Question 35)
PhD Student
University of South Carolina
Columbia, South Carolina
Physical Therapist
Proaxis Therapy
Greenville, South Carolina

Sue Falsone, PT, MS, SCS, ATC, CSCS, COMT (Questions 36, 37)
Owner, S&F: Structure and Function
Owner, Dr. Ma's Systemic Dry Needling
Head of Athletic Training and Sport Performance, United States Men's National Soccer Team
Phoenix, Arizona

Bryce W. Gaunt, PT, SCS (Questions 25, 28)
Clinical Director of Physical Therapy
Human Performance and Rehabilitation Center
St. Francis Rehabilitation Center, Main Campus
Columbus, Georgia

Josie L. Harding, BS, ATC, AT (Questions 11, 38)
Graduate Student, Athletic Training Program
A.T. Still University
Mesa, Arizona

Elizabeth E. Hibberd, PhD, ATC (Questions 2, 6, 33)
Assistant Professor
Director of the Athletic Training Research Laboratory
University of Alabama
Tuscaloosa, Alabama

Marilyn (Hintz) Kaminski, MS, ATC/L,CSCS (Question 38)
Efficient Movement
Creator of Abs Done Right
Owner/Clinician
Scottsdale, Arizona

Martin J. Kelley, PT, DPT, OCS (Question 29)
Clinical Education Facilitator, Advanced Clinician II
Good Shepherd Penn Partners/Penn Therapy & Fitness
Philadelphia, Pennsylvania

Joseph H. Kostuch, PT, SCS (Questions 25, 28)
Staff Physical Therapist
Human Performance and Rehabilitation Center
St. Francis Rehabilitation Center, Main Campus
Columbus, Georgia

Kevin Laudner, PhD, ATC, FACSM (Questions 3, 9)
Professor, School of Kinesiology and Recreation
Illinois State University
Normal, Illinois

Andréa Diniz Lopes, DSc (Questions 8, 18)
Postdoctoral Research Fellow in Clinical Outcomes Studies
A.T. Still University
Mesa, Arizona

Adam Lutz, PT, DPT (Questions 1, 17)
Physical Therapist, PhD student
Proaxis Therapy
Greenville, South Carolina

Lee N. Marinko, PT, ScD, OCS, FAAOMPT (Questions 15, 16)
Clinical Assistant Professor
Department of Physical Therapy and Athletic Training
Boston University College of Health and Rehabilitation Sciences: Sargent College
Boston, Massachusetts

Michael T. McKenney, MS, AT, CSCS (Question 26)
Assistant Professor/Clinical Coordinator
Athletic Training Program
Grand Canyon University
Phoenix, Arizona

Lori A. Michener, PhD, PT, ATC, SCS (Questions 10, 12)
Professor, Director of Clinical Outcomes, and Director of COOR Laboratory
Division of Biokinesiology and Physical Therapy
University of Southern California
Los Angeles, California

Joseph B. Myers, PhD, ATC (Questions 2, 6, 33)
Professor, Department of Exercise and Sport Science
Director, Human Movement Science Doctoral Curriculum
University of North Carolina at Chapel Hill
Chapel Hill, North Carolina

Thomas W. Nesser, PhD (Question 5)
Professor, Department of Kinesiology, Recreation, and Sport
College of Health, and Human Performance
Indiana State University
Terre Haute, Indiana

Jonathan K. Park, MD (Question 14)
Interventional Radiologist
Fellow and Clinical Instructor
David Geffen School of Medicine, University of California Los Angeles (UCLA
Los Angeles, California

Gail P. Parr, PhD, ATC (Questions 13, 36)
Professor, Department of Kinesiology
Towson University
Towson, Maryland

Brian J. Phillips, PT, DPT (Questions 25, 28)
Staff Physical Therapist
Human Performance and Rehabilitation Center
St. Francis Rehabilitation Center, Main Campus
Columbus, Georgia

Kelsey Picha, MS, ATC (Question 32)
Athletic Training Program
Arizona School of Health Sciences
A.T. Still University
Mesa, Arizona

Michael T. Piercey, PT, DPT, Cert. MDT, CMP, CSCS (Question 29)
Advanced Clinician I
Good Shepherd Penn Partners/Penn Therapy & Fitness
Philadelphia, Pennsylvania

Eric L. Sauers, PhD, ATC, FNATA (Questions 8, 18, 32)
Professor and Chair
Department of Interdisciplinary Health Sciences
Arizona School of Health Sciences
A.T. Still University
Mesa, Arizona

Aaron Sciascia, MS, ATC, NASM-PES (Questions 4, 7, 30)
Coordinator
Shoulder Center of Kentucky
Lexington, Kentucky

Michael A. Shaffer, PT, ATC, OCS (Questions 21, 22)
Coordinator for Sports Rehabilitation, UI Sports Medicine
Clinical Supervisor, UIHC Department of Rehabilitation Therapies
Institute for Orthopaedics, Sports Medicine and Rehabilitation
University of Iowa
Iowa City, Iowa

Ellen Shanley, PhD, PT, OCS (Questions 31, 35)
Clinical Research Scientist
Proaxis Therapy
Greenville, South Carolina
Director, Athletic Injury Research, Prevention and Education
SC Center for Rehabilitation and Reconstruction Sciences
Arnold School of Public Health
University of South Carolina
Columbia, South Carolina

Alison R. Snyder Valier, PhD, AT, FNATA (Question 19)
Associate Professor
Athletic Training Programs
A.T. Still University
Mesa, Arizona

Angela Tate, PT, PhD, Cert. MDT (Question 39)
Associate Faculty
Arcadia University
Glenside, Pennsylvania
Clinical Director
Willow Grove Physical Therapy
Willow Grove, Pennsylvania

Chuck Thigpen, PhD, PT, ATC (Questions 1, 17)
Clinical Research Scientist
Proaxis Therapy
Greenville, SC
Director, Program in Observational Clinical Research in Orthopedics
SC Center for Rehabilitation and Reconstruction Sciences
Adjunct Assistant Professor, Department of Physical Therapy
Arnold School of Public Health
University of South Carolina
Columbia, South Carolina
Assistant Consulting Professor, Doctor of Physical Therapy Division, Department of Orthopedics, Department of Community and Family Medicine
Duke University School of Medicine
Durham, North Carolina
Adjunct Assistant Professor, Clemson Bioengineering Department
Clemson University
Clemson, South Carolina

W. Steven Tucker, PhD, ATC (Question 34)
Associate Professor
Department of Kinesiology and Physical Education
University of Central Arkansas
Conway, Arkansas

Tim L. Uhl, PhD, ATC, PT, FNATA (Questions 24, 27)
Director of Musculoskeletal Laboratory
Professor, Athletic Training
University of Kentucky
College of Health Sciences
Lexington, Kentucky

Matthew K. Walsworth, MD, PT (Questions 12, 14)
Interventional and Diagnostic Radiologist
West Los Angeles Veterans Affairs Medical Center
Assistant Clinical Professor
David Geffen School of Medicine, University of California Los Angeles
Los Angeles, California

Preface

The Quick Questions series was developed to provide clinicians with brief, direct, actionable answers to clinical questions that they encounter in the daily practice of sports medicine to help optimize patient care. Today, information access is easier than it has ever been. However, it is a challenge to find the time and to develop the skill to consume and synthesize large bodies of evidence to distill knowledge into action. Because we typically do not have the time to complete this daunting task for every clinical question that arises, we often turn to our peers and colleagues for advice. One of the most trusted sources of information in health care is the expert consult. The Quick Questions series is like having a team of sports medicine experts with you on the sidelines or in the clinic to provide you with concise, straightforward advice to answer your most important clinical questions.

The editor of each book is a leading expert in his or her area of sports medicine practice who has assembled a team of expert clinicians and scholars to develop answers to 39 of the most commonly posed and clinically important questions. Each book is a compendium of expert advice from clinicians with the knowledge and experience to help guide your clinical decision making to provide safe and effective patient care.

In this book, *Quick Questions in the Shoulder: Expert Advice in Sports Medicine*, Dr. Kellie Huxel Bliven and her team of expert contributing authors have answered 39 of the most important clinical questions for one of the most complex joints of the human body that poses significant challenges for clinicians. This book begins with a series of fundamental questions pertaining to shoulder function, emphasizing the importance of posture, the hips and trunk, and strengthening. Next, the focus turns to the diagnosis of shoulder injuries, providing a wealth of information to assist clinicians in diagnosing injuries ranging from shoulder impingement to cervical radiculopathy. Subsequently, a section on injury treatment and rehabilitation provides expert advice on a broad range of areas such as choosing patient-rated outcomes measures, treating various conditions such as scapular dyskinesis, and determining when athletes can return safely to play following a brachial plexopathy. The final section of the book is dedicated to the overhead athlete and includes answers to a wide variety of questions such as screening measures, pitch count guidelines, return-to-throwing progressions, microinstability in tennis players, and training modifications for swimmers.

With the busy schedules, job stresses, and time constraints inherent to sports medicine practice, it is my sincere hope that this series proves to be a valuable resource full of expert advice that you find helpful in caring for your patients and athletes.

Eric L. Sauers, PhD, ATC, FNATA
Series Editor

Introduction

The complexity of shoulder injuries routinely presents challenges to clinicians. This book aims to answer many of the common questions pertaining to the athletic shoulder. The questions for this book were generated through dialogue with athletic trainers, physical therapists, and physicians working as clinicians, educators, and researchers in a variety of employment settings. The initial list of more than 70 clinical questions was categorized into common themes and relevance; it was then reduced to the 39 clinical questions presented in this book. The contributing authors, chosen for their expertise in shoulder research and/or clinical practice, were invited to write a response for a particular question using their content expertise, clinical judgments, and supporting evidence.

The questions are presented in 4 sections: (I) Factors Related to Shoulder Function; (II) Injury Diagnosis; (III) Injury Treatment and Rehabilitation; and (IV) The Overhead Athlete. Although the responses are not intended to be in-depth analyses of the available evidence, each question and response should provide the clinician with a quick understanding of the *what*, *when*, *why*, or *how* regarding many common questions about the athletic shoulder.

Kellie C. Huxel Bliven, PhD, ATC
Associate Professor, Kinesiology Program
College of Graduate Health Studies
A.T. Still University
Mesa, Arizona

SECTION I

FACTORS RELATED TO SHOULDER FUNCTION

QUESTION 1

What Factors Contribute to Forward Head and Rounded Shoulder Posture, and Why Is It Important to Assess?

Adam Lutz, PT, DPT and Chuck Thigpen, PhD, PT, ATC

Forward head and rounded shoulder posture (FHRSP) is a commonly observed deviation in posture, but its importance is not easily understood. Although often associated with patients with shoulder, neck, and interscapular pain, FHRSP is not consistently identified as a risk factor for pain. The ideal resting posture for the head and shoulder girdle is thought to be slightly anterior to the vertical plumb line that was long considered "normal." FHRSP is hypothesized to lead to muscle imbalances and alterations in optimal length-tension relationships that contribute to poor neuromuscular control of the upper quarter, abnormal scapulohumeral rhythm, scapular dyskinesis, abnormal muscle activation, and impaired strength.[1]

Posture is adaptive in nature and the result of habitual or repetitive positions and/or activities. As with all mechanical systems, changes in the resting position/posture of the human body effect changes in force production required for initiation of movement and for control of movement segments once initiated. FHRSP is regularly hypothesized to alter length-tension relationships of the upper quarter musculature. Common myofascial adaptations associated with FHRSP include

Huxel Bliven KC, ed. *Quick Questions in the Shoulder: Expert Advice in Sports Medicine* (pp 3-5).

shortening of the pectoralis minor; weakness and poor endurance of cervical extensors; increased activation of posterior cervical musculature, including the upper trapezius at rest and during movement; and adaptive lengthening and weakness of deep cervical flexors.[2,3] Many of these hypothesized adaptations associated with FHRSP are associated with neck and upper quarter pain.

FHRSP is thought to disrupt coordination and length-tension relationships, leading to decreased subacromial joint space via the altering of scapular function. Scapular function is classically described as scapulohumeral rhythm, which is the timing and rate of movement of the humerus to the scapula over the scapulothoracic junction. Normal scapulohumeral rhythm is hypothesized to maintain proper length-tension relationships and preserve subacromial joint space.

Scapular dyskinesis, which is examined further in subsequent chapters, is a common impairment identified in patients with neck, interscapular, and shoulder pain. Through alterations in optimal length-tension relationships, FHRSP is thought to contribute to scapular dyskinesis.[1] Scapular dyskinesis may be the cause of impairments in the upper quarter or a symptomatic response to another primary upper quarter pathology, but it is commonly observed in patients with shoulder impingement syndrome, labral injury, nerve injury, and multidirectional instability. Of note, resolution of shoulder impingement syndrome is not correlated with improvement to scapular kinematics. Although a lengthy discussion of scapular dyskinesis is not within the scope of this response, it is important to examine the scapular resting position and quality of movement in patients with FHRSP who present with neck, interscapular, or shoulder pain.

Kalra et al[4] found that acromiohumeral distance (AHD) was decreased in subjects with the arm elevated to 45 degrees with a "slouched" or "normal" posture when compared with an "upright" posture. They found no difference in subjects with rotator cuff disease (RCD) and asymptomatic subjects. That these AHD findings were insignificant between subjects with and without RCD is congruous with posture not consistently being identified as a risk factor for pain. Kebaetse et al[5] identified significant strength differences in the scapular musculature of individuals sitting in a slouched position when compared with those in a normal sitting posture, whereas similar strength differences have not been identified in individuals who only exhibit protracted and forward scapular positions.

Nontraumatic neck and upper quarter pain is often multifactorial in nature, with risk factors related to exposure and biomechanics, in addition to psychosocial and other confounding factors. While posture is associated with these risk factors, it appears that FHRSP is identified in conjunction with other impairments in the presence of pain. Repetitive or prolonged postural deviations in conjunction with repetitive upper quarter movements are commonly identified in individuals in industrial or factory settings who develop neck and upper quarter pain. Cervicothoracic or rib hypomobility and/or hypermobility combined with FHRSP likely also contribute to the development of neck and upper quarter pain; recent evidence suggests immediate pain relief of neck and/or upper quarter pain with manipulative interventions aimed at cervicothoracic segments and ribs.[6]

FHRSP is hypothesized to alter optimal length-tension relationships of the upper quarter musculature, which can change force production capabilities, potentially leading to impaired scapular kinematics and compensatory/substitution-based movement patterns that may predispose an individual to exposure- and biomechanical-based neck and upper quarter pain. With that said, evidence is limited on the importance of FHRSP as a direct contributor to neck and upper quarter pain. Although it has long been identified as an essential component of the musculoskeletal evaluation in patients with neck and upper quarter pain, it has never been identified as the primary impairment in individuals with symptomatic neck or upper quarter pain and dysfunction. Appropriate examination and evaluation of neck and upper quarter pain should always begin with a comprehensive history and should include an assessment of posture; however, the examination should continue with a thorough assessment of the neck and upper quarter so that the entire clinical picture becomes apparent and an appropriate, comprehensive intervention is established.

References

1. Thigpen CA, Padua DA, Michener LA, et al. Head and shoulder posture affect scapular mechanics and muscle activity in overhead tasks. *J Electromyogr Kinesiol.* 2010;20(4):701-709.
2. Grimmer K, Trott P. The association between cervical excursion angles and cervical short flexor muscle endurance. *Aust J Physiother.* 1998;44(3):201-207.
3. Hagberg M, Harms-Ringdahl K, Nisell R, Hjelm EW. Rehabilitation of neck-shoulder pain in women industrial workers: a randomized trial comparing isometric shoulder endurance training with isometric shoulder strength training. *Arch Phys Med Rehabil.* 2000;81(8): 1051-1058.
4. Kalra N, Seitz AL, Boardman ND III, Michener LA. Effect of posture on acromiohumeral distance with arm elevation in subjects with and without rotator cuff disease using ultrasonography. *J Orthop Sports Phys Ther.* 2010;40(10):633-640.
5. Kebaetse M, McClure P, Pratt NA. Thoracic position effect on shoulder range of motion, strength, and three-dimensional scapular kinematics. *Arch Phys Med Rehabil.* 1999;80(8): 945-950.
6. Strunce JB, Walker MJ, Boyles RE, Young BA. The immediate effects of thoracic spine and rib manipulation on subjects with primary complaints of shoulder pain. *J Man Manip Ther.* 2009;17(4):230-236.

QUESTION 2

How Does the Trunk Contribute to Upper Extremity Function and Injury Risk in Overhead Athletes?

Joseph B. Myers, PhD, ATC and
Elizabeth E. Hibberd, PhD, ATC

Clinicians commonly treat shoulder and elbow injuries in athletes who participate in overhead sports like baseball, softball, tennis, and swimming. Although the injury rates in these sports might be lower than in other sports that involve more body contact or collision, the time lost when injuries occur is significantly higher, and many times the injuries require surgery as part of the treatment.[1] During clinical evaluation of these injuries, a significant amount of time is afforded for the examination of the shoulder and elbow. However, the overhead motions associated with these arm injuries rely heavily on contributions from the trunk (hips, spine, and torso) to perform activity required to be successful during sport participation.

Motions like throwing, serving, and swimming strokes rely on the summation of speed principle, in which the speeds produced in the distal segments of the kinetic chain (the arm in this case) result from the sequence and speeds of proximal moving segments (in this case, the hips, lower torso, and upper torso of the trunk). Often, dysfunction in the trunk may contribute to the development of these injuries seen in overhead athletes, thus necessitating the trunk to be part of the injury

Huxel Bliven KC, ed. *Quick Questions in the Shoulder: Expert Advice in Sports Medicine* (pp 7-12).

evaluation. Ineffective transfer of energy from the trunk to the arm is generally thought to result in too much arm motion to compensate for the lack of proximal chain contribution, thus contributing to injury.

The following are 3 common ways that trunk motion and flexibility can contribute to dysfunction of the arm during overhead sport: faulty trunk posture, trunk inflexibility, and abnormal trunk motions during the overhead task. All 3 factors result in higher torques and forces on the upper extremity, which may cause injury.

Faulty Trunk Posture

Athletes who participate in overhead sports, especially swimmers, are notorious for having faulty posture. Typically, overhead athletes exhibit increased forward head and rounded shoulder posture, resulting in thoracic kyphosis (Figure 2-1). Faulty posture is believed to result from training and participation adaptations that include altered muscle lengths, increased muscle tightness, and strength imbalances. Overhead athletes often exhibit strong, tight anterior musculature (primarily pectoralis major and minor), with accompanying weakened, lengthened posterior musculature (scapular stabilizers).

These faulty posture characteristics can cause an interplay of factors including scapular dyskinesis, a narrowed subacromial space, decreased glenohumeral flexibility, and muscle strength imbalances, all of which are associated with the development of various shoulder impingements (primary, secondary, and internal impingement), rotator cuff tendinopathies, diffuse shoulder pain, and valgus extension overload elbow injuries in overhead athletes.

Because of the soft tissue contribution to faulty posture in overhead athletes, it appears that pectoral stretching and scapular stabilizer strengthening intervention programs are effective in restoring normal posture. Research has shown that individuals who perform 6 weeks of postural restoration exercises, such as resisted scapular retraction, shoulder shrugs, shoulder external rotation, and shoulder flexion exercises, and perform pectoral muscular stretching experience significant improvements in posture, scapular movement patterns, and glenohumeral mover and rotator cuff strength.[2,3] By improving posture, shoulder movement patterns, and strength, the risk of injury in overhead athletes should be reduced.

Trunk Inflexibility

During pitching, throwing, serving, and swimming, sequential rotation of the pelvis and upper torso creates a necessary rotational lag between the trunk segments, which contributes to momentum transfer across the trunk segment to the upper

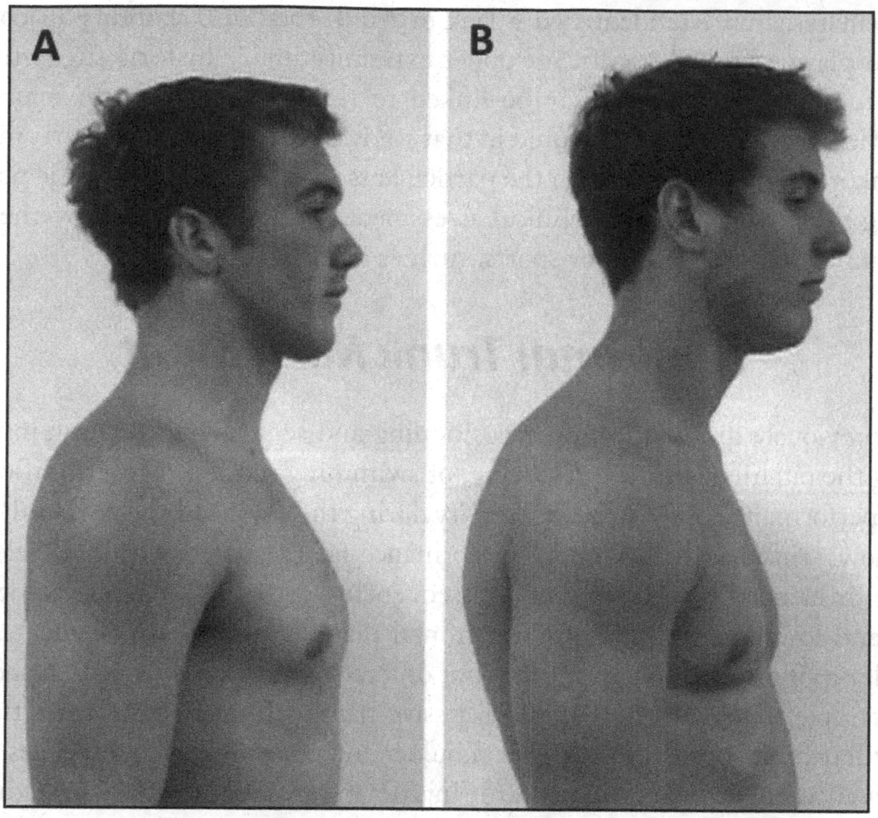

Figure 2-1. (A) Normal posture. (B) Forward head and rounded shoulder posture commonly exhibited in overhead athletes.

extremity via effective muscle force production through stretch-shortening contractions. The result is sequenced timing and force production by the upper extremity musculature, which optimizes athletic task performance.

Ineffective use of the trunk segment to transfer momentum and generate rotational momentum is thought to increase reliance on the upper extremity to make up for the loss of energy, thereby increasing the loads placed on the shoulder and elbow joints. Limited trunk rotation flexibility (ie, not having sufficient upper torso, lower torso, or hip flexibility) may be associated with upper extremity injuries in throwing athletes because it can interfere with the necessary sequential trunk rotation. In addition, after ball release in pitching/throwing, the torso rotates toward the intended target, helping to decelerate the throwing arm and minimizing the distraction forces experienced at the upper extremity joints. Therefore, restricted trunk rotation flexibility toward the direction of the throwing target may limit the ability of the trunk segment to contribute to arm deceleration, thereby leading to greater upper extremity joint load and risk of injury.

Recent research has identified a lack of trunk rotation flexibility in collegiate softball players with a significant upper extremity injury history, suggesting that trunk rotation inflexibility may be linked to throwing-related arm injury.[4] The trunk flexibility variables measured in that study were simple goniometric measures of trunk motion performed with the participants in various sport-specific positions, making them well suited for clinical assessment of trunk motion in overhead athletes and those who play other sports, such as golf.

Abnormal Trunk Movement

As previously discussed, proper positioning and sequencing of trunk movement during the pitching, throwing, serving, or swimming motion play a significant role in the performance of the upper extremity during the overhead sport tasks. Research has shown that baseball pitching performance (as measured with ball velocity) is highly influenced by the amount and sequencing of both transverse plane (upper torso and lower torso) rotations and frontal plane (trunk tilt) movements. These also play a significant role in the amount of forces and torques placed on the arm.[5,6] For example, pitchers who exhibit excessive trunk tilt away from their throwing arm will exhibit significantly higher shoulder and elbow forces and torques that are associated with throwing-related arm injury (Figure 2-2).[6] Thus, through proper instruction in appropriate trunk positions and movement patterns, performance can be improved while the injurious forces and torques on the upper extremity are reduced.

Similar to those in throwers, trunk position and movement during the swimming stroke contribute to both stroke performance and injury risk. For example, swimmers with a body roll angle during the recovery phase of the swim stroke that does not fall near the recommended 45 degrees of rotation can experience shoulder pain because this potentially contributes to the development of errors further in the stroke cycle. Excessive body roll angle can initiate a crossover entry position during both the recovery and pull-through phases and create impingement in the shoulder. Conversely, a lack of body roll during the recovery phase can increase mechanical stress on the shoulder, leading to improper hand entry position with a large angle of shoulder elevation and increased compressive forces of the subacromial shoulder structures.[7] As with throwing, addressing trunk position and movement through instruction may be a viable means to improve performance while reducing injury.

Injuries to the shoulder and elbow commonly occur in overhead athletes and often result in significant time loss from participation. While the injury occurs to the upper extremity, contributing factors to that injury may be present in

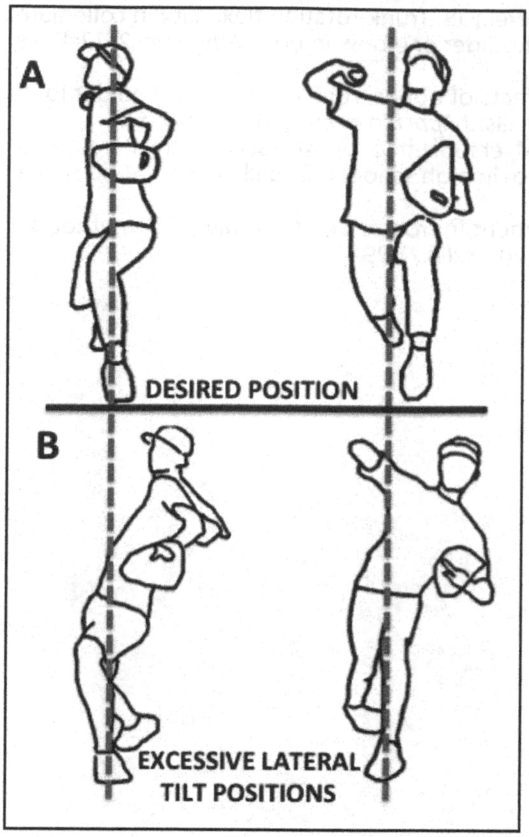

Figure 2-2. (A) Desired amount of lateral tilt during pitching. (B) Excessive lateral tilt during pitching, which results in increased forces and torques placed on the shoulder and elbow.

more proximal segments of the kinetic chain (hips, lower torso, and upper torso), thus requiring evaluation of these factors when setting injury-prevention and treatment goals. Contributing factors include faulty trunk posture, trunk inflexibility, and abnormal trunk motions during participation that result in high torques and forces being placed on the upper extremity. Fortunately for clinicians, these factors can typically be addressed through therapeutic exercise, which includes strength training, stretching, and technique instruction. The result is better overhead sport performance with a decrease in the stress and accompanying injury risk placed on the upper extremity during overhead sport.

References

1. Dick R, Sauers EL, Agel J, et al. Descriptive epidemiology of collegiate men's baseball injuries: National Collegiate Athletic Association Injury Surveillance System, 1988-1989 through 2003-2004. *J Athl Train.* 2007;42(2):183-193.
2. Kluemper M, Uhl TL, Hazelrigg H. Effect of stretching and strengthening shoulder muscles of forward shoulder posture in competitive swimmers. *J Sports Rehabil.* 2006;15(1):58-70.
3. Wang CH, McClure P, Pratt NE, Nobilini R. Stretching and strengthening exercises: their effect on three-dimensional scapular kinematics. *Arch Phys Med Rehabil.* 1999;80(8):923-929.

4. Aragon VJ, Oyama S, Oliaro SM, Padua DA, Myers JB. Trunk-rotation flexibility in collegiate softball players with or without a history of shoulder or elbow injury. *J Athl Train*. 2012;47(5): 507-513.
5. Aguinaldo AL, Buttermore J, Chambers H. Effects of upper trunk rotation on shoulder joint torque among baseball pitchers of various levels. *J Appl Biomech*. 2007;23(1):42-51.
6. Oyama S, Yu B, Blackburn JT, Padua DA, Li L, Myers JB. Effect of excessive contralateral trunk tilt on pitching biomechanics and performance in high school baseball pitchers. *Am J Sports Med*. 2013;41(10):2430-2438.
7. Yanai T, Hay JG, Miller GF. Shoulder impingement in front-crawl swimming: I. A method to identify impingement. *Med Sci Sports Exerc*. 2000;32(1):21-29.

QUESTION 3

Do Hip Mobility and Strength Affect Shoulder Function in Athletes?

Kevin Laudner, PhD, ATC, FACSM

The lower extremity plays an important role in the sequence of events necessary for various overhead functions, especially those in overhead sports, such as the volleyball spike, tennis serve, and overhead throwing motion. More specifically, the lower extremity is responsible for generating force production, and proper hip mobility is critical to facilitating transfer of forces from one segment to another along the kinetic chain proximally through the trunk, shoulder, elbow, wrist, and ultimately in the direction of whatever task is being performed. As such, deviations in the mobility and strength of the hip can have significant detrimental effects on the forces transmitted to the proximal segments, resulting in not only decreased athletic performance but also increased risk of injury.[1] Although these hip deviations can negatively affect any segment in the kinetic chain, the shoulder is often compromised because of its unstable nature.

The hips are a major force producer for various athletic motions, and overhead sports are no exception. Probably the biggest role of hip strength is that it produces a massive amount of force that is distributed throughout the kinetic chain during

Huxel Bliven KC, ed. *Quick Questions in the Shoulder: Expert Advice in Sports Medicine* (pp 13-16).

most overhead athletic motions and creates most of the power necessary for these athletic motions. Strength is also essential to ensure proper stride length, which aids in keeping these kinetic forces directed toward the intended target. This is especially critical in throwing sports (eg, baseball, softball, javelin throwing, and football passing). After the hips generate this power, the force is transmitted to the upper extremity, which aides in improving athletic performance by reducing the force production necessary from the shoulder, thereby reducing the risk of injury.

Although overall hip strength is necessary for good force production, there are some key hip motions that play a vital role in the process. More specifically, good hip abduction and extension strength of the trail leg (the leg on the same side as the throwing arm) assist in driving the body toward the intended target, generating massive amounts of force that are then transmitted to the upper extremity. This transfer of kinetic energy is made evident by the high positive correlation between increased leg push-off forces and increased arm and wrist velocities, which ultimately results in increased ball velocity.[2]

Force production is not the only benefit of good hip strength. Proper strength assists in stabilizing and aligning the pelvis, which creates a stable link for force transference between the lower and upper extremities. More specifically, hip abduction of the trail leg is necessary to prevent downward tilting of the ipsilateral pelvis, while the hip extensors of the lead leg (the leg on the opposite side of the throwing arm) eccentrically contract to stabilize the pelvis during hip flexion.[1] Improper positioning of the pelvis can disrupt this kinetic chain and result in extra and unnecessary force production by the shoulder. Over time, the accumulation of undue forces on the shoulder can result in microtrauma of the soft tissue structures. If untreated, this pathological cycle can continue until pain and injury develop. This is similar to what can occur with insufficient hip range of motion (ROM), which will be discussed next.

Although force production and stabilization are major responsibilities of the hips during overhead athletic motions, this force can be wasted if the distal segments are not optimally aligned with the proximal segments. An athlete's trunk follows the motion of his or her hips as he or she rotates toward the intended target.[3] As such, good hip mobility during the various overhead athletic movements allows for optimal pelvis orientation and, therefore, optimal positioning for transference of the generated lower extremity forces to the trunk and upper extremity.[4]

Hip rotation ROM is a critical characteristic necessary for transferring force throughout the kinetic chain. During the acceleration phase of the throwing motion, the lead foot should contact the ground with the toes pointed in the general direction of the intended target.[1] This task requires good hip external rotation of the lead leg and internal rotation of the trail leg hip.[5] Consider a baseball pitcher who has insufficient internal rotation ROM of the trail leg or insufficient external rotation of the lead leg. If the trail leg hip does not internally rotate enough, then the trunk of the pitcher may fail to align with the intended target, leaving the trunk rotated more toward the throwing arm side. This positioning can limit energy transfer and cause the pitcher to throw across his or her body, ultimately putting unnecessary stress on the shoulder.[1,3] Similarly, if the lead leg cannot externally rotate enough to align the trunk with the intended target at foot contact, then all the force developed by the hips and lower extremity is abruptly halted before the force can be transferred to the upper extremity. Both insufficiencies can ultimately lead to a disruption in the kinetic chain, thereby placing unnecessary stress on the shoulder in an effort to generate more force.[1,3] Insufficiencies in hip ROM can also affect athletic performance, resulting in, for example, decreased arm speed and ultimately decreased ball velocity among baseball players.[4]

Disruption of force transference can also occur among athletes with limited hip abduction, adduction, and extension ROM. These deficiencies primarily affect the athlete's stride length. During the throwing motion, the stride length varies based on the type of athletic motion but is typically slightly less than the athlete's height.[1,3] However, if the hips have insufficient abduction-adduction arc of motion, this distance can be dramatically reduced.[4] Once this occurs, all of the force that was developed in the hips and subsequent lower extremity is disrupted as the body moves toward the intended target. For example, picture your body falling forward. A long, sufficient stride allows for the forces developed as your body moves forward to continue in this direction. Conversely, if you were to abruptly put your foot down as you were falling forward, similar to what happens with a short stride, a sudden disruption of that forward motion occurs. When this happens in an overhead sport activity such as throwing, this disruption of the lower extremity forces developed would then place an increased demand on the motion and forces necessary in the shoulder.

Because of the large forces produced and flexibility necessary in the hips for proper kinetic energy transference, alterations in these characteristics can have significant negative effects on the shoulder, creating undue additional stress. Over time, the accumulation of this additional stress can cause soft tissue damage and result in time lost from competition. Therefore, it is important for clinicians to assess and address hip strength and ROM deficiencies to assist in the prevention, evaluation, and treatment of various shoulder pathologies.

References

1. Wilk K, Meister K, Fleisig GS, Andrews JR. Biomechanics of the overhead throwing motion. *Sports Med Arthrosc Rev.* 2000;8(2):124-134.
2. MacWilliams BA, Choi T, Perezous MK, Chao EY, McFarland EG. Characteristic ground-reaction forces in baseball pitching. *Am J Sports Med.* 1998;26(1):66-71.

3. Dillman CJ, Fleisig GS, Andrews JR. Biomechanics of pitching with emphasis upon shoulder kinematics. *J Orthop Sports Phys Ther.* 1993;18(2):402-408.
4. Robb AJ, Fleisig G, Wilk K, Macrina L, Bolt B, Pajaczkowski J. Passive ranges of motion of the hips and their relationship with pitching biomechanics and ball velocity in professional baseball pitchers. *Am J Sports Med.* 2010;38(12):2487-2493.
5. Tippett SR. Lower extremity strength and active range of motion in college baseball pitchers: a comparison between stance leg and kick leg. *J Orthop Sports Phys Ther.* 1986;8(1):10-14.

QUESTION 4

Can Core Strength and Stability Improve Upper Extremity Function?

Aaron Sciascia, MS, ATC, NASM-PES

It has long been hypothesized that physical function is best achieved when core strength and stability are optimized. This concept can be applied to both the upper and lower extremities; however, it may be more critical for appreciating upper extremity physical function such as in overhead throwing or lifting tasks. Overhead activities require the shoulder to be exposed to and sustain repetitive loads. The segmental activation of the body's links, known as the kinetic chain, allows this to occur effectively. Proper muscle activation is achieved through the generation of energy from the central segment (ie, the core). The energy must be transferred to the terminal links of the shoulder, elbow, and hand for overhead tasks to be executed. The kinetic chain is best characterized by the following 3 components: optimized anatomy, reproducible efficient motor patterns, and the sequential generation of forces. However, anatomical or physiological deficits, such as weakness and/or tightness in the core musculature or altered core stability, can lead to deleterious effects in the shoulder. An appreciation of the role of core strength and stability in kinetic chain function and of how the usage of kinetic chain–based

Huxel Bliven KC, ed. *Quick Questions in the Shoulder: Expert Advice in Sports Medicine* (pp 17-21).

rehabilitation will improve upper extremity physical function will assist the clinician in overcoming existing deficits.

The core includes numerous foundational components, including the vertebral column, rib cage, hips, pelvis, and proximal lower limbs. It is composed of a multitude of muscles within the central portion of the human body, and all the muscles have individual actions that also collectively work together for dynamic stabilization and force generation. For dynamic tasks to be optimally executed, the muscles must provide segmental spinal stability for local trunk strength and balance, which in turn allows the extremities to produce a desired output.

Two terms that are at times interchanged but actually have different meanings are *core strength* and *core stability*. Core strength is the physiological capability of the centralized muscles to generate force. Conversely, core stability is the ability to control the position and motion of the trunk over the pelvis and leg to allow optimum production, transfer, and control of force and motion to the terminal segment in integrated kinetic chain activities.[1] The kinetic chain model is routinely used as a framework to describe the manner in which the individual body segments interact with each other to perform a dynamic task, especially tasks specific to the upper extremity (ie, overhead throwing). For example, to effectively throw a ball overhead, force is developed in the legs and trunk in a closed-chain fashion, is funneled through the scapulohumeral complex using closed-chain biomechanics, and is transferred to the arm. By definition, then, a kinetic chain is a coordinated sequencing of activation, mobilization, and stabilization of body segments to produce a dynamic activity.[2]

The concept of having optimized core strength and stability as a requirement for optimized upper extremity function has been popular for many years.[1,3] It has been suggested that a lack of core strength and/or stability (called kinetic chain breakage) places the upper extremity at risk for injury because the stability and force-generation capabilities of the core create altered loads on the tissues of the arm. Recent investigations have indeed found that the presence of core instability, as determined through decreased single-leg balance performance, negatively affects arm function[4] and is more prevalent in individuals with shoulder pain.[5] These findings support the idea that shoulder function is dependent on the function of the segments that precede it in regard to overhead tasks.

Subscribing to the kinetic chain model of function, the logical assumption would be that improvement of common deficiencies within the core (immobility of the pelvis, hip, and/or trunk; muscular weakness of the same areas; and alterations in muscle recruitment and timing) would decrease the risk of injury to the upper extremity. However, to date, no comparative studies have been performed to determine whether upper extremity performance improves after the application of core stability or strength interventions. As a result of the lack of hard evidence, clinicians are left to disseminate biomechanical data and anecdotal clinical phenomena in an attempt to describe a relationship between core strength and/or stability and the occurrence of upper extremity injury.

To effectively enhance kinetic chain function and reduce injury risk to the arm, it must be understood that focusing solely on core strength and stability is an incomplete method of management. Just as improvements in scapular function do not directly reduce the incidence of injury to the shoulder, improvements in core function do not directly reduce the incidence of injury either. Because core function is one of many pieces that should be appreciated, clinicians should attempt to integrate the improved core with the performance of shoulder-specific tasks to maximize usage of the kinetic chain. Kinetic chain enhancement through rehabilitation can be accomplished when clinicians target 3 key components for maximizing kinetic chain function. First, all segments within the kinetic chain (in addition to the core segments) should be free from anatomical injury and have optimal physiological function. Next, the development of efficient task-specific motor patterns for task execution should be encouraged. Once the motor patterns have been established, clinicians can attempt to minimize the redundancy in the motor system for maximal efficiency.[2]

Kinetic chain–based upper extremity rehabilitation requires enhancements to be made to a deficient core, but the enhancements should serve as the foundation for what is known as integrated rehabilitation. Integrated rehabilitation utilizes core function in which the legs, hips, and trunk drive the arm throughout specific movements. Although the prescription of core strengthening and stabilization exercises is beyond the scope of this chapter, the concept of integrated movements is illustrated in basic maneuvers such as the low row (Figure 4-1) and more complex maneuvers such as fencing (Figure 4-2). Ideally, time should be dedicated toward first developing core strength and stability (optimizing anatomy), then integrating the newly developed core function with shoulder tasks (well-developed motor patterns), and finally progressing the individual to complex tasks. This process adequately directs and educates the motor system to perform optimally (reducing redundancy in the motor system). The latter component is important in the clinical progression; improvements in strength and stability may lead to altered performance initially, because the individual is not familiar with how to use the new gains. Clinicians should allot adequate time to retrain the motor system to perform under the new degrees of freedom or constraints.

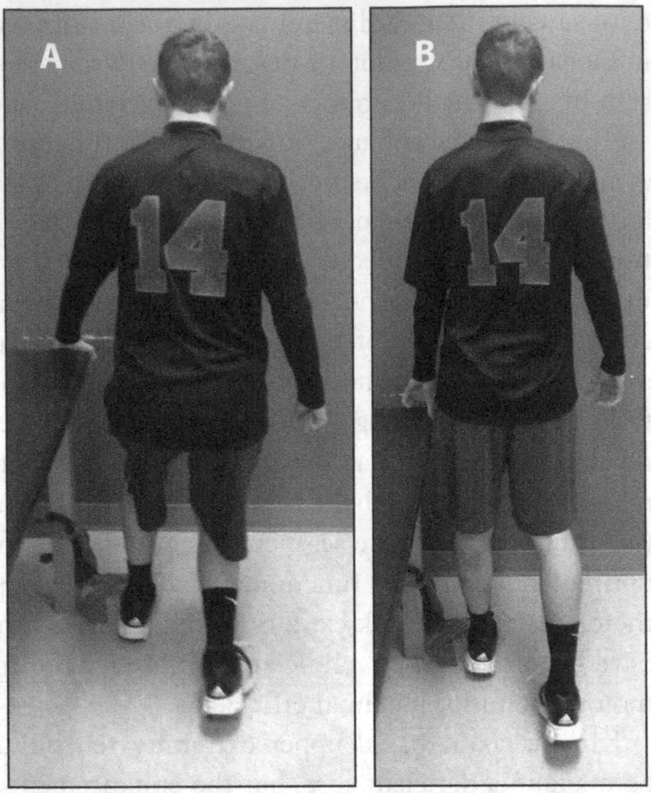

Figure 4-1. (A) The low row exercise, which helps facilitate scapular retraction, is performed standing with the knees flexed and grasping a firm, immovable surface. (B) The patient is instructed to extend the legs while simultaneously extending the arm, pushing back against the grasped surface.

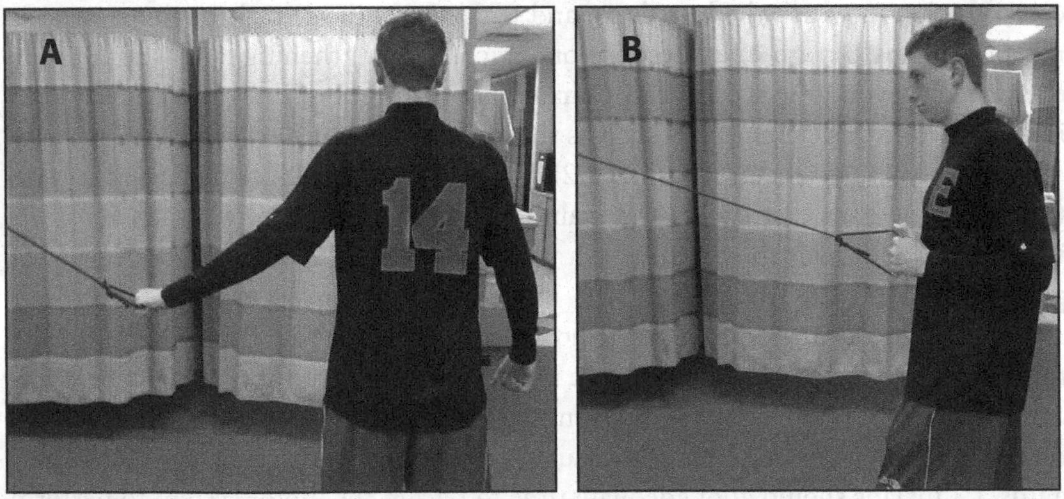

Figure 4-2. The fencing maneuver uses multiple kinetic chain segments to enhance proper muscle scapular muscle activation. (A) The patient is asked to begin with the arm slightly abducted and then (B) to retract the scapula and adduct the arm while rotating the trunk.

References

1. Kibler WB, Press J, Sciascia A. The role of core stability in athletic function. *Sports Med.* 2006;36(3):189-198.
2. Sciascia A, Thigpen C, Namdari S, Baldwin K. Kinetic chain abnormalities in the athletic shoulder. *Sports Med Arthrosc.* 2012;20(1):16-21.
3. Hibbs AE, Thompson KG, French D, Wrigley A, Spears I. Optimizing performance by improving core stability and core strength. *Sports Med.* 2008;38(12):995-1008.
4. Radwan A, Francis J, Green A, et al. Is there a relation between shoulder dysfunction and core instability? *Int J Sports Phys Ther.* 2014;9(1):8-13.
5. Reeser JC, Joy EA, Porucznik CA, Berg RL, Colliver EB, Willick SE. Risk factors for volleyball-related shoulder pain and dysfunction. *PM R.* 2010;2(1):27-36.

QUESTION 5

What Are Appropriate Weight Training Exercises to Avoid Shoulder Pain and Discomfort?

Thomas W. Nesser, PhD

Shoulder pain during resistance training is fairly common, but it can and should be avoided. The risk of injury during resistance training can be minimized by ensuring that exercises are completed using proper technique.

One strategy for avoiding shoulder pain is the use of dumbbells rather than a barbell. A barbell keeps the hands in a fixed position and does not allow the arms to move through their natural range of motion. Such an action can adversely stress the joints and cause shoulder pain. Using a dumbbell allows the arm to move naturally through the range of motion and also promotes dynamic stabilization of the smaller rotator cuff muscles by requiring greater balance and stability with a more open-chain exercise. As such, the amount of weight used will be less with dumbbells than with a barbell.

The overhead press (Figure 5-1) is a common exercise for targeting shoulder musculature. The trunk and legs stabilize the weight as the shoulders, upper chest, and arms press the weight overhead. The setup for this exercise includes grip and feet shoulder-width apart. The dumbbells or bar is placed high on the chest; the

Huxel Bliven KC, ed. *Quick Questions in the Shoulder: Expert Advice in Sports Medicine* (pp 23-27).

Figure 5-1. (A) Overhead press start/down position. (B) Overhead press end/up position.

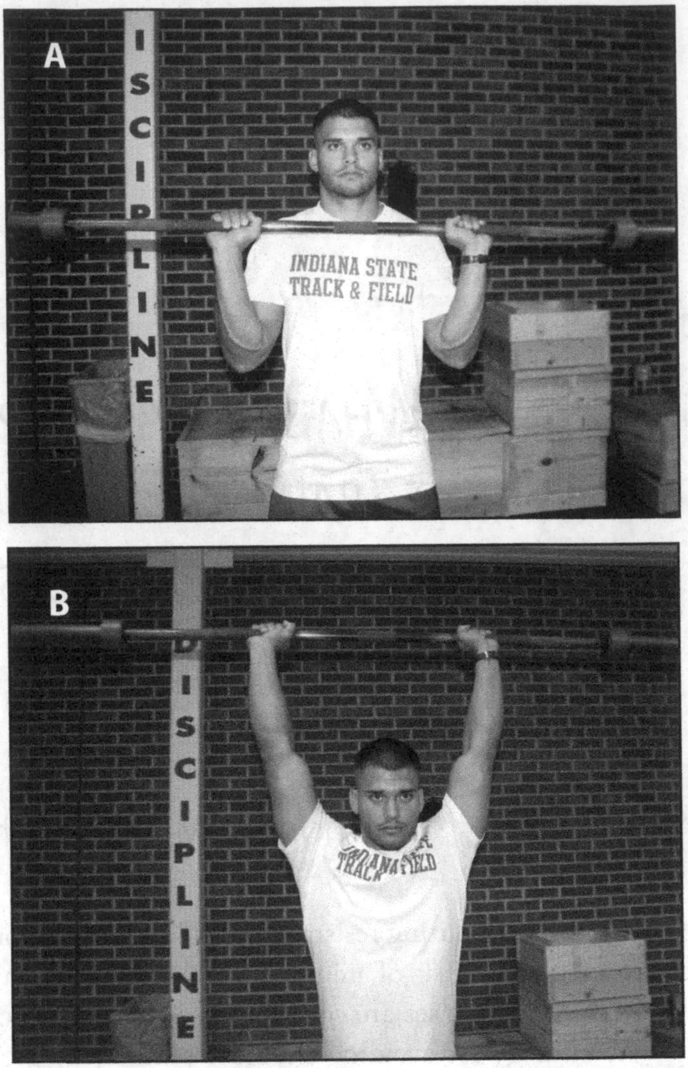

chest should be held up and the elbows should face forward and be slightly in front of the dumbbell or bar. During the lift, the individual should look forward; the act of looking up can put adverse stress on the neck. The dumbbell or bar should be pressed in a straight line over the head, which requires the head to be tilted slightly back so the dumbbell or bar does not contact the chin or nose. As the dumbbell or bar clears the forehead, the torso must be shifted forward as the dumbbell or bar is pressed overhead. The back should be kept straight. The movement should continue until the elbows are locked. The dumbbell or bar is then returned back to the starting point. This exercise requires both balance and strength. If done incorrectly, it can easily result in an unstable position that increases the chances for injury. Common errors in performing this exercise include failing to keep the eyes looking forward and moving the head to watch the bar; allowing the elbows

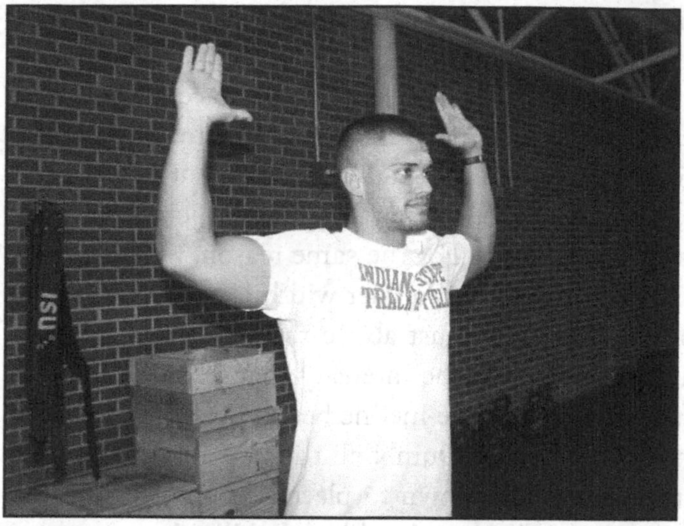

Figure 5-2. High-five position that athletes should avoid during an overhead press lift.

to flare out to a wide position, referred to as a high-five position (Figure 5-2); and leaning backward instead of keeping the back straight. These errors individually or collectively can have adverse effects on the shoulders, neck, and back. Although it is an excellent exercise for increasing shoulder strength, this exercise should not be part of the early regimen in shoulder rehabilitation.

The lat pull-down requires the use of several joints and is typically performed using a bar-and-pulley system. If done properly, it can increase the strength of the latissimus dorsi, muscles in the upper back, and biceps. Proper technique includes keeping the chest tall and leaning slightly from the hips to take pressure off the lower back. Keeping the elbows facing forward, the athlete pulls the bar to the upper chest and then returns it to the starting position. Similar to the overhead press, failing to keep the elbows facing forward can place the shoulders in a compromising position (ie, anterior glide of the shoulder).[1] A variation of this exercise is to pull the bar behind the neck. However, this option is not advisable because it decreases the range of motion performed, compromises the effectiveness of the exercise, and potentially places adverse stress on the neck and shoulders.

Pull-ups are an exercise with basically the same movement as the lat pull-down. The difference is that the body is pulled toward the bar (hands) rather than pulling the bar toward the body. When performing the pull-up, the bar should come to the front of the shoulders. It is important to begin the exercise by contracting the scapular stabilizers and latissimus dorsi to stabilize the scapulae in retraction. This movement can be practiced by hanging from a bar and pulling the body toward it using only the scapular muscles. If it is performed correctly, the body will only move a few inches.

The upright row can be used to strengthen shoulder musculature, but it should be used with extreme caution because it is known to cause shoulder pain. There are no known variations of this exercise that minimize shoulder discomfort; consequently, it should be avoided in most instances.[2]

The bench press is a common exercise for the chest but can place considerable stress on the anterior shoulders if performed incorrectly. In performing the exercise, the elbows should remain close to the body and not flared out to the side. Similar to the overhead press, this position opens up the shoulder joint, reducing stability and increasing susceptibility to injury. For the same reason, a wide grip is not recommended[1-3]; rather, slightly wider than shoulder width is appropriate. The dumbbell or bar should be lowered to a point just above the xiphoid process. In performing the bench press, it is typically not the intensity that leads to shoulder pain but the use of inappropriate technique.[1] The incline bench press is a potential alternative strategy for reducing shoulder pain. Dumbbell flies are another exercise for the chest. Unfortunately, this exercise is known to place adverse stress on the shoulders. As such, it too is not recommended in a shoulder rehabilitation program.[2]

The back squat, although not a shoulder exercise, can put considerable stress on the shoulders. The back squat can be completed with the dumbbell or bar in a high or low position. The high position places the dumbbell or bar at the base of the neck, and the low position places the dumbbell or bar across the posterior deltoid and middle trapezius. Because the low position opens the shoulder joints farther, it can cause discomfort. Moving the dumbbell or bar into the high bar position may resolve the problem. In addition, stress on the shoulders can be reduced by keeping the elbows pointing down and contracting the muscles of the upper back. An alternative form of this exercise is to move the barbell to the front of the shoulders and complete a front squat.[2]

Lateral raises can be a safe and effective means for strengthening shoulder musculature, and varying the amount of weight can target different muscles (eg, deltoid, rotator cuff).[2] The exercise can be performed from a seated or standing position. While holding the torso straight and stationary, dumbbells should be held with the palms of the hands facing toward the body. The dumbbells are lifted laterally (abduction) with a slight bend in the elbow. The motion should continue until the arms are parallel to the floor. This action will engage the deltoid muscle if higher weights are used and recruit the supraspinatus if lower weights and a 45-degree elevation position are used, and it will not place harmful stress on the shoulders. The dumbbells should be lowered slowly to the starting position. Because of the relatively short length of the deltoids and the long length of the arms, minimum load is necessary to train the muscle.

The use of weight machines may or may not cause shoulder pain. Machines move in a fixed position. Similar to the use of a barbell, the arms are often not allowed to move through a natural range of motion, thus placing undue stress on the shoulders. However, machines can be set to limit range of motion, allowing an individual to avoid positions that lead to pain.

Overall, shoulder pain during resistance exercise can be common, but one strategy for avoiding pain is to focus on technique. If proper technique still results in shoulder pain, the exercise should be avoided.

References

1. Kolber MJ, Beekhuizen KS, Cheng MS, Hellman MA. Shoulder injuries attributed to resistance training: a brief review. *J Strength Cond Res.* 2010;24(6):1696-1704.
2. Durall CJ, Manske RC, Davies GJ. Avoiding shoulder injury from resistance training. *Strength Cond J.* 2001;23(5):10-18.
3. Fees M, Decker T, Snyder-Mackler L, Axe MJ. Upper extremity weight-training modifications for the injured athlete. A clinical perspective. *Am J Sports Med.* 1998;26(5):732-742.

SECTION II

INJURY DIAGNOSIS

QUESTION 6

What Are the Most Common Forms of Shoulder Impingement in Athletes, and How Can One Differentiate Between Them?

Elizabeth E. Hibberd, PhD, ATC and
Joseph B. Myers, PhD, ATC

During overhead activities, high, repetitive stresses are placed on the glenohumeral joint, often leading to overuse injuries. To counteract these repetitive stresses, the glenohumeral joint relies heavily on dynamic stability provided by the shoulder musculature. Dynamic stability is accomplished through the combined contractions of the rotator cuff musculature, the long head of the biceps, and other muscles surrounding the glenohumeral joint such as the deltoids and pectoral muscles. When the stresses involved in the overhead motion exceed the capability of the muscular system to control these stresses, overuse injury can result. A common injury-producing scenario for the overhead athlete includes the combination of high stresses at the shoulder that are repeatedly applied to normal tissues, eventually resulting in tissue attenuation and failure. This can be referred to as acquired repetitive microtrauma. This repetitive microtrauma can cause various shoulder impingement syndromes, which present as pain, loss of range of motion, and decreased strength and function, and can be especially debilitating to overhead

Huxel Bliven KC, ed. *Quick Questions in the Shoulder: Expert Advice in Sports Medicine* (pp 31-38).

athletes. Shoulder impingement syndrome can be classified as external or internal impingement.

Types of Impingement

External impingement is the compression of the rotator cuff by the undersurface of the acromion and can be classified as primary or secondary. Primary external impingement is irritation of the rotator cuff caused by extracapsular stresses in the subacromial space. These causes include subacromial spurring and an altered shape of the acromion. These bony deformities affect the amount of space available in the subacromial space and increase the incidence of impingement. A type 1 acromion is flat and has a low incidence of impingement; type 2 is curved and has a greater incidence of impingement; and type 3 is beaked and has the highest incidence of impingement.[1] Tendinopathy occurs as the rotator cuff thickens as a result of continual irritation. Tendinopathy and associated tears in individuals with primary external impingement most commonly occur in older athletes. Radiographs can confirm the diagnosis of primary external impingement. Treatment of primary external impingement is typically subacromial decompression surgery before the weaknesses and decreased range of motion of the rotator cuff can be addressed.

Secondary external impingement is the inability to keep the humeral head centered in the glenoid cavity during movement because of shoulder instability created by rotator cuff weakness or a loose shoulder joint capsule or ligament. Secondary external impingement is also called subacromial impingement syndrome and is a mechanical compression of the rotator cuff, biceps tendon, or subacromial bursa by the acromion (Figure 6-1). During movement, the humeral head narrows the subacromial space, leading to increased compression of the structures within the subacromial space. Functional narrowing of the subacromial space can occur as a result of weak rotator cuff and scapular stabilizing muscles, altered scapular kinematics caused by weak scapular stabilizing musculature, abnormal posture, and posterior shoulder tightness. With this functional narrowing, impingement of the supraspinatus, long head of the biceps, and the subacromial bursa may occur. The other rotator cuff muscles, the infraspinatus, teres minor, and subscapularis, are also susceptible to being impinged as they become confluent with the glenohumeral capsule. Compression of any of these structures may lead to pain and dysfunction, especially in an overhead athlete. Secondary external impingement is more likely to occur in younger athletes, who will report anterior shoulder pain as the primary symptom. The treatment goal for an individual with secondary external impingement is to address the underlying instability, which can often be done with an effective strengthening and stretching program.

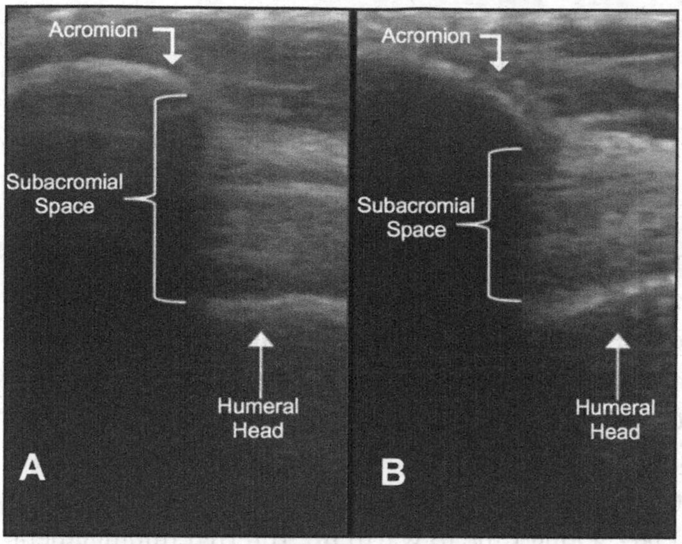

Figure 6-1. Subacromial space ultrasound images showing (A) normal subacromial space distance and (B) decreased subacromial space distance leading to increased mechanical compression.

Internal impingement, or posterior-superior glenoid impingement, occurs as a result of contact between the articular side of the supraspinatus or infraspinatus tendon and the posterosuperior glenoid rim, which leads to undersurface rotator cuff wear and fraying of the glenoid labrum.[2] Primary internal impingement is caused by humeral retrotorsion, which is an osseous adaptation that is characterized by the twisting of the proximal physis of the humerus due to the forces and long-axis torques associated with throwing. Overhead athletes have been identified to have greater humeral retrotorsion on the dominant limb than on the nondominant limb, suggesting that bilateral variations are influenced by the degree of upper extremity activity.[3] Increased humeral retrotorsion is of interest because it has been shown to contribute to decreased internal rotation and increased external rotation range of motion of the throwing arm and may contribute to the development of internal impingement.[3]

Secondary internal impingement that results from anterior instability and scapular dyskinesia causing repetitive contact between the greater tuberosity of the humeral head and the posterosuperior aspect of the glenoid is the most common cause of posterior shoulder pain in the overhead athlete. During the overhead throwing motion, the anterior capsule is exposed to high tensile stress, with the arm in external rotation with abduction, which leads to gradual stretching of the capsular collagen over time, and that leads to increased anterior capsular laxity. This laxity may manifest as anterior instability or microinstability, which allows the humeral head to translate anteriorly during the overhead motion, causing the posterior rotator cuff musculature to be impinged on the posterosuperior glenoid rim.

The repetitive nature of throwing may cause fatigue of the posterior rotator cuff muscles and cause alterations in scapular movement, and it may place more stress on the posterior capsule to maintain joint stability. The distractive stress will cause repetitive microtrauma to the posterior capsule and a fibroblastic healing response, resulting in hypertrophy and contracture. In one study, athletes with pathologic internal impingement exhibited significantly greater posterior capsule tightness on the dominant side than on the nondominant side, when seen in contrast with healthy control subjects.[4] This tight and hypertrophied posterior capsule causes a shift in the arthrokinematics of the glenohumeral joint. Tightness of the posterior capsule, which is known to limit glenohumeral internal rotation, can create anterior and superior humeral translations during flexion that cause impingement of the supraspinatus or infraspinatus tendon and the posterosuperior glenoid rim.

With internal impingement, pain is felt in the posterior shoulder. Athletes may report feeling stiff and that it takes a long time to warm up. Internal impingement has been described in 3 progressive stages. In stage 1, the primary complaint is stiffness and shoulder pain that occurs during the overhead throwing motion even after a prolonged warm-up; stage 2 is made up of similar symptoms with a progressive increase in posterior joint line pain and subluxation of the humeral head; and stage 3 is characterized as the failure of conservative treatment to improve symptoms.[5] Conservative treatment includes rest, ice, use of nonsteroidal anti-inflammatory drugs, internal rotation stretching, and periscapular musculature and rotator cuff strengthening. Surgical intervention may be used if conservative treatments do not improve symptoms.

Although many of the symptoms of these different impingement syndromes may present in similar manners, proper diagnosis is imperative to provide the most effective treatment to the individual. A summary of special tests for external (subacromial) and internal (posterior-superior glenoid) impingement is provided in Table 6-1. These special tests have been shown to have good sensitivity and/or specificity and are useful when diagnosing impingement syndromes. In addition to these special tests, glenohumeral range of motion and muscle strength tests should be used in developing a targeted intervention program to help the injured athlete.

Table 6-1

Special Tests for Impingement Evaluation

External (Subacromial) Impingement

Special Test	*Testing Position*	*Positive Test*	*Diagnostic Values*[6]
Cross-body adduction test	Patient is seated with the shoulder flexed to 90 degrees. The examiner passively adducts the arm horizontally across the body.	Pain with horizontal adduction, indicating compression of structures in the subacromial space.	Sensitivity: 75% Specificity: 61%
Drop arm sign	The patient is seated with his or her shoulder maximally abducted. The patient then slowly lowers the arm to 90 degrees of abduction. If he or she is able to maintain this position, slight overpressure is provided to the wrist by the examiner.	Inability to maintain the arm in 90 degrees of abduction or weakness when overpressure is provided, indicating supraspinatus tear.	Sensitivity: 45% to 73% Specificity: 70% to 77%
Empty can (Jobe) test	Patient is seated with the arm in the scapular plane (90 degrees of flexion with approximately 30 degrees of horizontal abduction), with the shoulder internally rotated so the thumb is pointing down. The examiner applies a downward force on the distal end of the humerus while the patient resists the pressure.	Pain during the test and/or inability or weakness when resisting the pressure, indicating impingement of the supraspinatus.	***Pain*** Sensitivity: 52% Specificity: 33% ***Weakness*** Sensitivity: 50% to 52% Specificity: 67% to 87% ***Pain or weakness*** Sensitivity: 74% Specificity: 30%

(continued)

Table 6-1 (continued)

Special Tests for Impingement Evaluation

External (Subacromial) Impingement

Special Test	*Testing Position*	*Positive Test*	*Diagnostic Values*[6]
External rotation resistance	Patient is seated with the elbow flexed to 90 degrees in neutral rotation. The examiner applies a medially directed force to the wrist (attempting to cause internal rotation), while the patient is instructed to resist the pressure and maintain the neutral rotation of the shoulder.	Pain during the test and/or inability or weakness when resisting the pressure, indicating impingement of structures in the subacromial space, primarily the teres minor and infraspinatus.	***Pain*** Sensitivity: 33% to 56% Specificity: 87% to 90% ***Weakness*** Sensitivity: 55% Specificity: 25%
Hawkins-Kennedy test	Patient is seated with the shoulder and elbow flexed to 90 degrees. The examiner passively internally rotates the shoulder at a variety of degrees of horizontal adduction.	Pain with internal rotation, indicating compression of structures in the subacromial space.	Sensitivity: 63% to 74% Specificity: 40% to 89%
Scapular reposition test	If a patient has positive Neer, Hawkins-Kennedy, Jobe, or painful arc test, the test is repeated while the examiner applies an anteriorly directed force on the scapula with the thenar eminence on the spine of the scapula and the forearm on the medial border of the scapula, moving the scapula into greater posterior tilting, external rotation, and retraction.	Pain is relieved and/or strength increases when the scapula is repositioned, indicating altered scapular kinematics causing functional narrowing of the subacromial space during movement.	Not applicable

(continued)

Table 6-1 (continued)

Special Tests for Impingement Evaluation

External (Subacromial) Impingement			
Special Test	***Testing Position***	***Positive Test***	***Diagnostic Values***[6]
Neer impingement sign	Patient is seated and the examiner passively flexes the shoulder maximally or until pain is felt.	Pain with flexion, especially between 60 and 120 degrees of flexion, indicating compression of structures in the subacromial space.	Sensitivity: 54% to 81% Specificity: 10% to 95%
Painful arc test	Patient is seated and actively abducts the arm to his or her maximal range of motion and then slowly lowers the arm back to the side of the body.	Pain with flexion, especially between 60 to 120 degrees of flexion, indicating compression of structures in the subacromial space.	Sensitivity: 49% to 75% Specificity: 33% to 80%
Internal (Posterior-Superior Glenoid) Impingement			
Special Test	***Testing Position***	***Positive Test***	***Diagnostic Values***[7]
Posterior impingement sign	Patient is seated and the elbow is flexed to 90 degrees while the shoulder is passively abducted 90 degrees, extended 10 degrees, and maximally externally rotated by the examiner.	Increase in posterior shoulder pain, indicating impingement of the posterior-superior glenoid labrum and/or the supraspinatus or infraspinatus tendon.	Sensitivity: 76% to 95% Specificity: 85% to 100%
Relocation test for impingement	Patient is supine and the elbow is flexed to 90 degrees while the shoulder is passively abducted 90 degrees, extended 10 degrees, and maximally externally rotated by the examiner, while the examiner places posterior pressure on the humeral head.	Posterior shoulder pain is relieved with the pressure, indicating abnormal kinematics that prevent the humeral head from remaining centered, leading to internal impingement.	Not applicable

References

1. Bigliani LU, Levine WN. Subacromial impingement syndrome. *J Bone Joint Surg Am.* 1997;79(12):1854-1868.
2. Walch G, Liotard JP, Boileau P, Noel E. Postero-superior glenoid impingement. Another shoulder impingement [in French]. *Rev Chir Orthop Reparatrice Appar Mot.* 1991;77(8):571-574.
3. Myers JB, Oyama S, Goerger BM, Rucinski TJ, Blackburn JT, Creighton RA. Influence of humeral torsion on interpretation of posterior shoulder tightness measures in overhead athletes. *Clin J Sport Med.* 2009;19(5):366-371.
4. Myers JB, Laudner KG, Pasquale MR, Bradley JP, Lephart SM. Glenohumeral range of motion deficits and posterior shoulder tightness in throwers with pathologic internal impingement. *Am J Sports Med.* 2006;34(3):385-391.
5. Jobe CM. Superior glenoid impingement. *Orthop Clin North Am.* 1997;28(2):137-143.
6. Hegedus EJ, Goode AP, Cook CE, et al. Which physical examination tests provide clinicians with the most value when examining the shoulder? Update of a systematic review with meta-analysis of individual tests. *Br J Sports Med.* 2012;46(14):964-978.
7. Meister K, Buckley B, Batts J. The posterior impingement sign: diagnosis of rotator cuff and posterior labral tears secondary to internal impingement in overhand athletes. *Am J Orthop (Belle Mead NJ).* 2004;33(8):412-415.

QUESTION 7

What Are the Best Clinical Tests for Determining if a Patient Has Scapular Dyskinesis and if It Is Contributing to His or Her Shoulder Pain and Dysfunction?

Aaron Sciascia, MS, ATC, NASM-PES

Altered scapular motion and altered position during motion have been termed *scapular dyskinesis*.[1] The definition of dyskinesis is the alteration of normal scapular kinematics. "Dys" (alteration of) "kinesis" (motion) is a general term that reflects loss of normal control of scapular motion. An alternative term that is often used interchangeably is *dyskinesia*. Dyskinesia is usually applied to abnormal active (voluntary) movements mediated by neurologically controlled factors. The scapular rotations (upward/downward rotation, anterior/posterior tilt, and internal/external rotation) are accessory motions, which by definition are involuntary in nature. The scapular translations can be performed voluntarily, but there are times when the scapula translates during arm motion without conscious consideration from the individual person. In addition to these motion distinctions, there are many other factors that can cause the altered scapular position and motion, such as bony injury (clavicle fractures, acromioclavicular joint separations), soft tissue disruption

Huxel Bliven KC, ed. *Quick Questions in the Shoulder: Expert Advice in Sports Medicine* (pp 39-43).

(scapular muscle detachments), and internal derangement (labral injury, compromised capsular tissue). Therefore, the more inclusive term *dyskinesis* is preferred.

Dyskinesis by itself is not an injury or a musculoskeletal diagnosis. In some instances, the visible winging of the scapula can have neurological roots, such as long thoracic nerve or accessory nerve palsies. Any suspicion of nerve involvement is best ruled out by diagnostic nerve conduction studies. In most cases, scapular dyskinesis should be viewed as a physical impairment similar to patellar tracking alterations seen in the knee. This must be fully understood by clinicians, because approaching scapular dyskinesis as a pathological entity can misguide treatment protocols and lead to less-than-optimal rehabilitation outcomes.

Under the classification of a physical impairment, scapular dyskinesis is best identified through observational analysis. Early attempts at assessment were focused on classifying the severity of abnormal scapular movement and position based on comparisons between the involved and noninvolved arms. The initial observational analysis described 4 types of dyskinesis (Type I—inferior angle prominence; Type II—medial border prominence; Type III—superior angle prominence; and Type IV—normal, symmetrical motion). These determinations were made by standing behind the patient with the patient's back exposed and asking the patient to elevate the arms overhead 3 consecutive times. The dyskinesis would be observed in the descent phase of the arm motion. Recent kinematic assessments have shown that more than one type of dyskinesis occurs simultaneously during arm motion.[2] As a result of these findings, it is now most appropriate to use a simple "yes" (dyskinesis present) or "no" (dyskinesis not present) assessment if any of the following observations are made: clinical observation of the medial and inferior scapular borders for winging or medial border prominence, lack of a smooth coordinated movement depicted as early scapular elevation or shrugging during ascending arm forward flexion, and rapid downward rotation during arm lowering from full flexion. A refined method consisting of observational analysis, which includes the use of 3- to 5-lb weights held by the patient during the overhead motion (performed up to 10 consecutive times), and the yes/no determination being made has been found to be both valid and reliable.[3,4] This method of assessment, called the scapular dyskinesis test, rates each arm individually and is the preferred means of determining whether scapular dyskinesis is present in patients with shoulder injury.[1]

To aid clinicians in confirming whether the observed alteration in scapular motion is clinically related to the shoulder dysfunction, additional maneuvers are available. It is possible that alterations of scapular motion are compensatory strategies to avoid stress on pain-sensitive tissue.[1] Therefore, clinicians can employ symptom-alteration maneuvers, also known as corrective maneuvers, to determine whether scapular dysfunction is contributing to the shoulder pain.

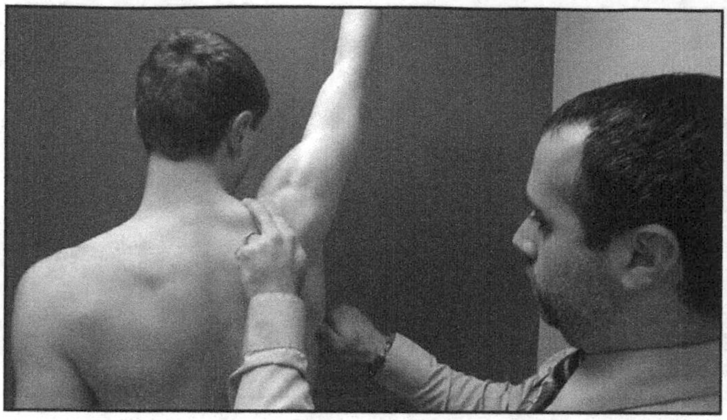

Figure 7-1. The scapular assistance test (SAT). The examiner assists serratus anterior and lower trapezius muscle activity as the arm is elevated. Improved arm elevation and relief of impingement symptoms indicate a positive test.

The first maneuver is known as the scapular assistance test (SAT).[1] The SAT involves manually assisting scapular upward rotation during shoulder elevation and determining the effect on pain. The patient is asked to elevate the involved arm as far as possible into forward flexion. The examiner then places one hand on the inferior angle and one hand on the superior border (Figure 7-1). The patient is asked to repeat the arm elevation with the addition of the examiner assisting the scapula during the elevation task. The result is positive when the active arm elevation range improves and/or pain with elevation is either decreased or abolished during the assisted maneuver. This test has demonstrated acceptable levels of reliability. It was later modified by incorporating scapular posterior tilting as well.

The second maneuver is known as the scapular retraction test (SRT).[1] This test was developed to illustrate to both the clinician and patient that strength loss in shoulder elevation may be caused by a loss of proximal stability of the scapular stabilizers rather than local stabilizers (ie, the rotator cuff muscles). Identifying the correct source of weakness is critical for the development of optimal shoulder rehabilitation regimens and for improving rehabilitation outcomes. The SRT is performed by first manually muscle testing the involved arm in 90 degrees of elevation, similar to the traditional manual muscle tests for the supraspinatus (Figure 7-2A). The examiner then manually stabilizes the scapula by placing a hand over the superior aspect of the shoulder and the forearm over the medial border of the scapula (Figure 7-2B). The muscle test is repeated, with a positive result being noted when the patient demonstrates a reduction of pain or an increase in shoulder elevation strength when the scapula is stabilized during isometric arm elevation in the scapular plane at 90 degrees. The SRT was later modified and termed the *scapular reposition test*, which involves manually positioning and stabilizing the medial border of the scapula with simultaneous posterior tilting in a slightly retracted position on the thorax.[5]

The observational and corrective maneuvers are designed to identify the presence of scapular dyskinesis and the potential role of scapular dysfunction on shoulder

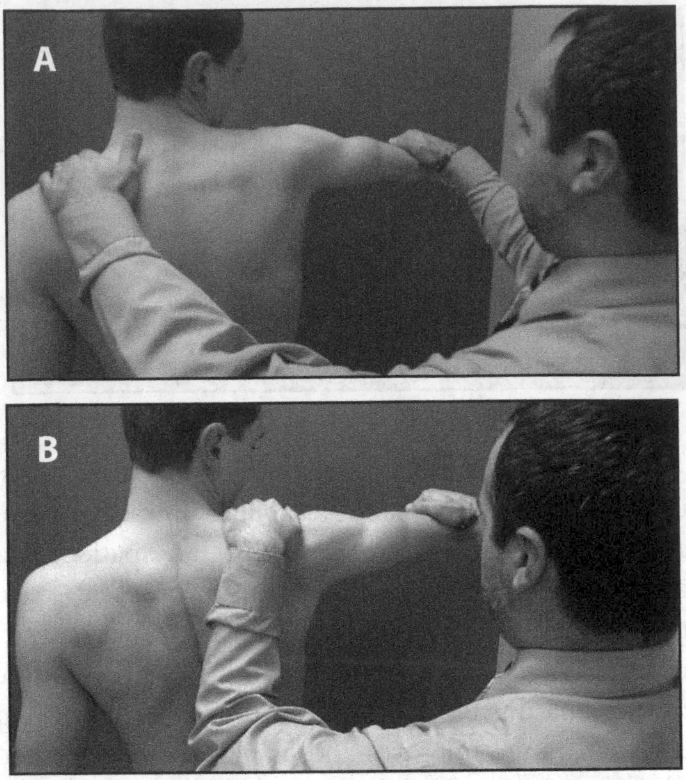

Figure 7-2. The scapular retraction test (SRT). (A) Following the performance of a standard manual muscle test, (B) the examiner stabilizes the medial scapular border and reapplies the muscle test. Improved demonstrated manual muscle test strength indicates a positive test.

pain. The major kinematic result of the corrective maneuvers is an increase in scapular upward rotation and posterior tilt (SAT) and/or scapular external rotation and posterior tilt (SRT), so a positive result indicates that rotator cuff strengthening is not necessary and the focus should be on rhomboid strengthening and serratus function in retraction. Although these tests are not capable of diagnosing a specific form of shoulder pathology, a positive SAT or SRT result shows that scapular dyskinesis is directly involved in producing the symptoms and indicates the need for inclusion of early scapular rehabilitation exercises to improve scapular control. A comprehensive shoulder examination is advocated, in which the traditional components of the physical examination should be employed to identify other impairments, including muscle weakness, strength imbalance, and/or motion alterations and to rule in or rule out identifiable shoulder pathology. It is recommended that clinicians attempt to resolve the shoulder and/or scapular dysfunction with conservative rehabilitation methods in the event that scapular dyskinesis is identified as being present and confirmed with the corrective maneuvers. However, if symptoms persist despite attempts at resolving scapular dysfunction and there are indicators that internal derangement is present, referral to an orthopedic surgeon may be warranted.

References

1. Kibler WB, Ludewig PM, McClure PW, Michener LA, Bak K, Sciascia AD. Clinical implications of scapular dyskinesis in shoulder injury: the 2013 consensus statement from the 'Scapular Summit.' *Br J Sports Med.* 2013;47(14):877-885.
2. Uhl TL, Kibler WB, Gecewich B, Tripp BL. Evaluation of clinical assessment methods for scapular dyskinesis. *Arthroscopy.* 2009;25(11):1240-1248.
3. McClure P, Tate AR, Kareha S, Irwin D, Zlupko E. A clinical method for identifying scapular dyskinesis, part 1: reliability. *J Athl Train.* 2009;44(2):160-164.
4. Tate AR, McClure P, Kareha S, Irwin D, Barbe MF. A clinical method for identifying scapular dyskinesis, part 2: validity. *J Athl Train.* 2009;44(2):165-173.
5. Tate AR, McClure PW, Kareha S, Irwin D. Effect of the scapula reposition test on shoulder impingement symptoms and elevation strength in overhead athletes. *J Orthop Sports Phys Ther.* 2008;38(1):4-11.

QUESTION **8**

What Is the Clinical Importance of Visual Scapular Dyskinesis in Overhead Athletes With Shoulder Symptoms?

Andréa Diniz Lopes, DSc and Eric L. Sauers, PhD, ATC, FNATA

Shoulder pain is reported frequently among athletes performing repetitive overhead activity. Normal scapular motion is required to maintain optimal muscle length-tension relationships, the subacromial space, and glenohumeral stability during overhead activity. As the arm is raised, the generally accepted pattern of scapular motion is upward rotation, posterior tilt, and external rotation along with clavicular elevation and retraction. Altered scapular motion is a common clinical problem and has been associated with a variety of shoulder disorders, such as rotator cuff disease, labral injury, and instability. However, altered scapular motion is also frequently observed in asymptomatic shoulders, and the presence of scapular motion asymmetry has been found to be equal between groups with symptomatic and asymptomatic shoulders. Clinical decision making is hindered, because the contribution of altered scapular motion to shoulder disability remains unclear. For instance, should overhead athletes who present with visual alterations in scapular motion during preseason screening be placed on a preventive program? Or, how

Huxel Bliven KC, ed. *Quick Questions in the Shoulder: Expert Advice in Sports Medicine* (pp 45-48).

does scapular winging contribute to shoulder pathology in overhead athletes with impingement symptoms?

Visual alterations in static scapular position and dynamic scapular motion have been termed *scapular dyskinesis*.[1] It can be multifactorial, and the dyskinesis may be either a cause or the result of pathology. So, it is important to evaluate and address each individual's specific impairments. Theoretically, scapular dyskinesis is the primary cause that results in shoulder dysfunction, an associated condition that contributes to injury causation, or an adaptive condition that arises to compensate for other dysfunction. However, the relationship between scapular dyskinesis and shoulder symptoms is not clear. In the case of primary scapular pathology, such as a nerve injury, it is clear that the injury creates the dyskinesis, which in turn affects shoulder function and can lead to shoulder pain. In cases such as impingement syndrome, labral injury, and instability, the dyskinesis may be causative, creating pathomechanics that predispose the arm to such injuries. Alternatively, the dyskinesis may be a response to injury, creating adaptive pathomechanics that increase the existing dysfunction.

Altered scapular position and/or motion, termed *scapular dyskinesis*, can be observed during weighted arm elevation using the scapular dyskinesis test (SDT).[2,3] The SDT is a reliable and valid method for detecting the presence of scapular dyskinesis during clinical evaluation of the shoulder.[2,3] Scapular motion is classified as normal, subtle, or obvious dyskinesis, based on the clinically observed scapular motion. Different patterns of scapular dyskinesis include scapular winging and/or dysrhythmia in the quality or quantity of scapular motion. Scapular winging occurs when the medial border and/or inferior angle of the scapula is posteriorly displaced away from the thorax. Dysrhythmia occurs when the scapula demonstrates premature or excessive elevation or protraction or non-smooth or stuttering motion during the concentric or eccentric phases of arm elevation. Those "subtypes" of scapular dyskinesis can be identified in isolation or together in the same athlete and in the concentric and/or eccentric phase of arm elevation. However, observational clinical assessment of scapular motion during arm elevation in patients, particularly athletes, can be challenging because of the multiple possible altered scapular motions and overlying musculature. Practice is needed to identify scapular dyskinesis and its different types of patterns that can be visually identified in patients during arm elevation.

In asymptomatic baseball players, studies have consistently shown that the throwing shoulder exhibits greater scapular upward rotation.[4] This may be an adaptation to overhead throwing that serves to spare the subacromial space. Baseball players with pathologic internal impingement have demonstrated less upward rotation and greater posterior tilting during arm elevation in the scapular plane than have asymptomatic athletes.[5] Furthermore, collegiate overhead throwing athletes with obvious scapular dyskinesis, identified using the SDT, exhibited less upward rotation, less clavicular elevation, and greater clavicular protraction than those with normal motion. However, there was no relationship between the presence of pain and scapular dyskinesis in these athletes.[3]

A prospective study of high school baseball players evaluated the role of scapular dysfunction identified using the SDT during preseason screenings to see if the presence of scapular dyskinesis was predictive of increased throwing-related injuries.[6] There were only 12 subsequent throwing injuries, and there were no differences in injury rates between baseball players with scapular dyskinesis (subtle or obvious) identified at preseason and those with normal scapular motion. The authors concluded that the presence of scapular dyskinesis in asymptomatic baseball throwers is not predictive of future shoulder or elbow injury.[6] This is consistent with the recommendations of the 2013 Scapular Summit, which state that alterations in scapular motion in athletes should be treated only if they are present in association with upper extremity injury.[1] However, side-to-side evaluation should be done to check for abnormal asymmetries because it has been demonstrated that throwing athletes have specific compensations in scapular position.

Scapular upward rotation was measured in collegiate swimmers with and without shoulder pain before and after a typical swimming practice, and a decrease was found in upward rotation following practice in the athletes with shoulder pain. This finding suggested that fatigue may have resulted in a loss of upward rotation and may have contributed to secondary impingement-type pain. However, the authors did not report whether these subjects had visually detectable scapular dyskinesis.

The limited studies of scapular motion in overhead throwing athletes suggest that increased scapular upward rotation is a healthy adaptive change in the dominant shoulder that is lost in athletes with scapular dyskinesis and internal impingement, and that swimmers with painful shoulders lose scapular upward rotation during a normal swimming practice. Collectively, these studies support the importance of normal scapular motion and muscular endurance to healthy shoulder function in overhead athletes.

Scapular dyskinesis may directly cause, contribute to, or be a result of shoulder symptoms in overhead athletes, and the presence of scapular dyskinesis in symptomatic athletes may limit athletic participation. Careful evaluation using the SDT is required to identify scapular dyskinesis in overhead athletes with shoulder symptoms. Patient-specific rehabilitation programs should be developed to correct scapular dyskinesis when it is associated with injury. Currently, it is not clear to what extent the presence of visual scapular dyskinesis contributes to disability in overhead athletes; future studies are warranted. It is recommended that symptomatic overhead athletes be tested for the presence of scapular dyskinesis and, if found, that a focused rehabilitation program aimed at restoring coordinated scapular motion, soft tissue mobility, and muscular endurance be implemented. Because of the limited data regarding the predictive importance of scapular dyskinesis for future injury, it is recommended that asymptomatic overhead athletes be screened for the presence of visual scapular dyskinesis and, if found, that these athletes be placed on a preventative strengthening and flexibility program to improve scapular motion and endurance.

References

1. Kibler WB, Ludewig PM, McClure PW, Michener LA, Bak K, Sciascia AD. Clinical implications of scapular dyskinesis in shoulder injury: the 2013 consensus statement from the 'Scapular Summit.' *Br J Sports Med.* 2013;47(14):877-885.
2. McClure P, Tate AR, Kareha S, Irwin D, Zlupko E. A clinical method for identifying scapular dyskinesis, part 1: reliability. *J Athl Train.* 2009;44(2):160-164.
3. Tate AR, McClure P, Kareha S, Irwin D, Barbe MF. A clinical method for identifying scapular dyskinesis, part 2: validity. *J Athl Train.* 2009;44(2):165-173.
4. Seitz AL, Reinold M, Schneider RA, Gill TJ, Thigpen CA. No effect of scapular position on 3-dimensional scapular motion in the throwing shoulder of healthy professional pitchers. *J Sport Rehabil.* 2012;21(2):186-193.
5. Laudner KG, Myers JB, Pasquale MR, Bradley JP, Lephart SM. Scapular dysfunction in throwers with pathologic internal impingement. *J Orthop Sports Phys Ther.* 2006;36(7): 485-494.
6. Myers JB, Oyama S, Hibberd EE. Scapular dysfunction in high school baseball players sustaining throwing-related upper extremity injury: a prospective study. *J Shoulder Elbow Surg.* 2013;22(9):1154-1159.

QUESTION 9

What Are the Best Clinical Tests for Measuring Posterior Shoulder Tightness, and How Should Results Be Used to Make Treatment Decisions?

Kevin Laudner, PhD, ATC, FACSM

The deceleration phase of various overhead sports, such as the throwing motion, tennis service, and volleyball spike, place a tremendous amount of force on the posterior shoulder. The accumulation of these repetitive forces can cause subsequent thickening of the posterior glenohumeral capsule and shortening of the posterior shoulder musculature.[1] Such soft tissue adaptations can cause further alterations in shoulder range of motion (ROM), which typically present as decreased internal rotation and horizontal adduction. Furthermore, athletes who accumulate these types of forces while still skeletally immature can also present with bony adaptions that alter ROM.[1,2] Although increased retroversion is believed to be beneficial for athletes, because it reduces stress to the anterior soft tissue restraints, posterior soft tissue adaptations have been repeatedly associated with shoulder pathology.[1,2] Therefore, the accurate assessment of posterior shoulder soft tissue tightness is critical in the prevention, diagnosis, and treatment of various shoulder injuries.

The first step in assessing posterior shoulder tightness is attempting to determine whether the tightness is caused by soft tissue alterations, bony alterations,

Huxel Bliven KC, ed. *Quick Questions in the Shoulder: Expert Advice in Sports Medicine* (pp 49-53).

Figure 9-1. Example of pathologic GIRD using 10% of total arc of motion method.

Total arc = 160°

10% x 160° = 16°

Pathologic GIRD = >16°

or both. However, without access to advanced diagnostic equipment, such as diagnostic ultrasonography, this is no easy task. The difficulty arises because both increased humeral retroversion and posterior soft tissue shoulder tightness can cause decreases in glenohumeral internal rotation ROM. However, increased humeral retroversion has been reported to increase glenohumeral external rotation ROM and cause a concomitant decrease in internal rotation, thereby leaving the total arc of motion (sum of total internal and external rotation) similar to that of the noninvolved shoulder.[2] As such, if bilateral differences do exist in the total arc of motion, these differences are most likely results of soft tissue, rather than bony, adaptations and should be measured and documented for treatment.

Although there are several methods of measuring posterior shoulder tightness, the gold standard is assessment of glenohumeral horizontal adduction ROM. Many clinicians will mistakenly simply measure glenohumeral internal rotation ROM and compare bilaterally. This bilateral difference has been termed *glenohumeral internal rotation deficit* (GIRD). However, as previously stated, this loss of internal rotation could stem from increased humeral retroversion, which cannot be treated. Although there is a distinct lack of consensus, some clinicians have reported classifications of GIRD to assist in determining the likelihood of injury. Pathologic GIRD has been defined as any difference greater than 25 degrees, with the acceptable level being approximately 20 degrees.[1] Some clinicians have also recommended comparing the total arcs of motion bilaterally, indicating that any difference in GIRD greater than 10% of the total arc of motion is pathological.[1] An example of this theory can be viewed in Figure 9-1. In this example, if the total arc of motion on the involved side is 160 degrees, then 10% would be 16 degrees. Based on this example, any bilateral difference in internal rotation (GIRD) of greater than 16 degrees would be considered pathological. However, subsequent studies have reported even smaller levels of GIRD and bilateral differences in the total arc of motion to increase the risk of injury, so these values should be used with caution.[2]

To avoid some of the misconceptions and pitfalls of measuring internal rotation ROM solely as a determinant of posterior shoulder tightness, many clinicians choose to measure glenohumeral horizontal adduction ROM. Although this motion also has a correlation with humeral retroversion, it is a very weak relationship, and therefore it can be used with more confidence than measurement

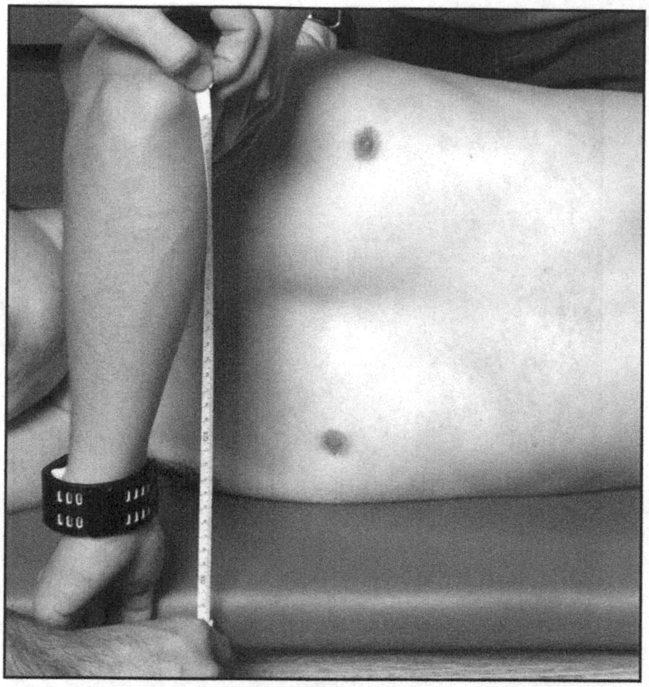

Figure 9-2. Side-lying method of measuring posterior shoulder tightness.

of internal rotation ROM. However, there are variations in the techniques used to measure this ROM. Some clinicians measure horizontal adduction motion with the patient side lying and the acromia aligned perpendicular to the examination table.[3] An examiner then manually stabilizes the scapula in a retracted position and moves the test side humerus into horizontal adduction. At the end ROM, a second examiner measures the distance from the patient's involved-side medial epicondyle to the examination table surface (Figure 9-2). A longer distance indicates more posterior shoulder tightness. Conversely, a shorter distance indicates less posterior shoulder tightness. However, positioning of the patient for this measurement is critical, as any forward or backward torso rotation will produce inaccurate results. Furthermore, a patient with a longer humerus will naturally have a shorter distance to the examination table than a patient with a shorter humerus, thus making comparison between patients difficult.

Because of the risk of inaccuracies when measuring glenohumeral horizontal adduction ROM in a side-lying position, this technique was later slightly modified to improve accuracy.[4] For this new measurement, the patient is placed in a supine position. The scapula is then secured by an examiner with application of a posterior force against the anterior portion of the scapula (Figure 9-3). The shoulder is then moved into passive horizontal adduction until the end ROM. In this position, a digital inclinometer (a standard goniometer can also be used) is aligned with the shaft of the humerus (Figure 9-4) to determine the angle between the humerus and a vertical reference. If the humerus were able to move past the vertical

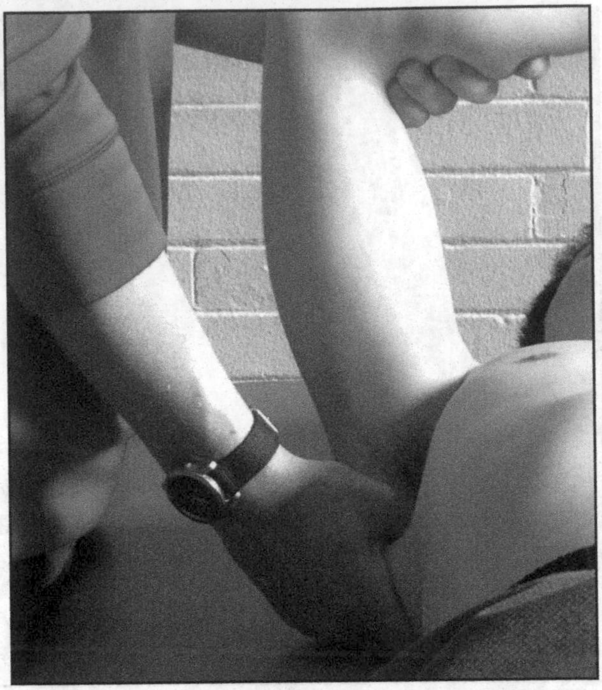

Figure 9-3. Stabilization of the scapula for supine measurement of posterior shoulder tightness.

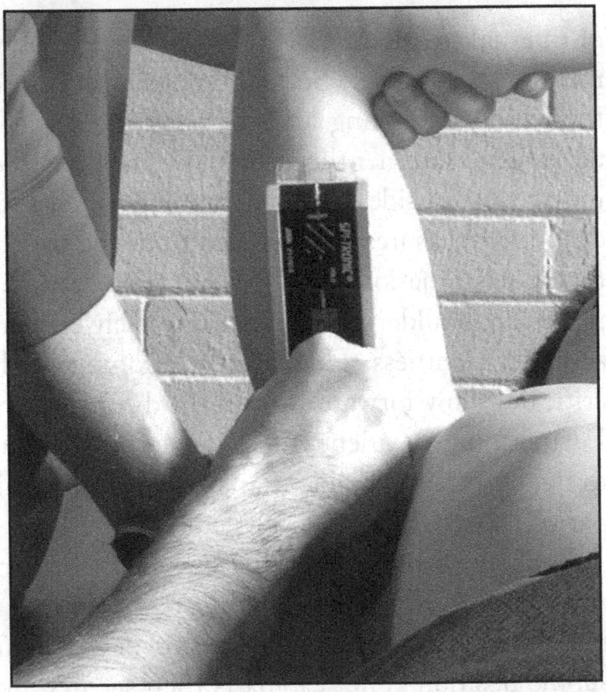

Figure 9-4. Digital inclinometer being used to measure the angle of the humerus relative to vertical reference for measuring posterior shoulder tightness.

reference point (ie, humerus is closer to the patient's body), then the motion would be increasing. Conversely, and what is often observed in the dominant arm of overhead athletes because of posterior shoulder tightness, the patient will be unable to even get the humerus to perpendicular (ie, humerus is further away from the body).

Although no pathological values have been determined for the supine horizontal adduction measurement technique, the throwing arm of baseball players typically presents with approximately −8 to 0 degrees of motion.[4] Again, this negative value means the humerus is not able to horizontally adduct to a vertical position (0 degrees) relative to the treatment table. Conversely, the nonthrowing arm of these athletes typically presents with approximately 5 to 10 degrees of motion.[4] Because of the strong association between posterior shoulder tightness and various shoulder and elbow injuries,[1,2] individuals who have flexibility values less than those in these ranges should be encouraged to complete a stretching and manual therapy program. Specific interventions may include various passive stretches, such as the sleeper stretch and passive glenohumeral horizontal adduction, as well as muscle energy technique and posterior glenohumeral joint mobilization.

Research has supported using a supine glenohumeral horizontal adduction ROM measurement to quantify posterior shoulder tightness. Because of the strong association between posterior shoulder tightness and various shoulder and elbow pathologies, this technique should be used in the prevention and treatment of such injuries.

References

1. Burkhart SS, Morgan CD, Kibler WB. The disabled throwing shoulder: spectrum of pathology. Part I: pathoanatomy and biomechanics. *Arthroscopy.* 2003;19(4):404-420.
2. Kibler WB, Kuhn JE, Wilk K, et al. The disabled throwing shoulder: spectrum of pathology—10-year update. *Arthroscopy.* 2013;29(1):141-161 e126.
3. Tyler TF, Roy T, Nicholas SJ, Gleim GW. Reliability and validity of a new method of measuring posterior shoulder tightness. *J Orthop Sports Phys Ther.* 1999;29(5):262-269; discussion 270-274.
4. Laudner KG, Stanek JM, Meister K. Assessing posterior shoulder contracture: the reliability and validity of measuring glenohumeral joint horizontal adduction. *J Athl Train.* 2006;41(4): 375-380.

QUESTION 10

Which History and Physical Examination Diagnostic Tests Can Confirm and Screen Superior Labral Anterior-to-Posterior Lesions?

Lori A. Michener, PhD, PT, ATC, SCS

Glenohumeral labral lesions are a common injury in athletes participating in overhead sporting activities. One type of labral lesion is the superior labral anterior-to-posterior (SLAP) lesion. Snyder et al[1] described a classification for the following 4 types of SLAP lesions: Type I, fraying and degeneration of the superior labrum with a normal biceps anchor; Type II, labral fraying with a detachment of the labrum and the biceps anchor from the superior glenoid; Type III, bucket-handle tear of the labrum with an intact biceps tendon insertion; and Type IV, a bucket-handle tear of the labrum that extends into the biceps. Type I SLAP lesions are not considered a frequent source of shoulder pain or symptoms, whereas Type II through IV SLAP lesions can give rise to symptoms and functional limitations. More recently, the Snyder classification was modified to include 9 categories to more specifically describe the locations, such as the glenohumeral ligaments, of injury and other associated anatomical tissue pathology.

Huxel Bliven KC, ed. *Quick Questions in the Shoulder: Expert Advice in Sports Medicine* (pp 55-58).

Mechanistically, a SLAP lesion may be caused by repetitive overhead throwing. The repetitive placement of the shoulder into abduction with excessive external rotation loads the labrum and long head of the biceps tendon and may lead to injury. In addition, eccentric force applied via the biceps-labral complex to the labrum during the throwing motion may cause labral injury. A SLAP lesion may also be induced traumatically with a fall on an outstretched hand.

SLAP lesions may or may not cause shoulder pain. If pain is present, it typically presents in the region of the SLAP lesion (superior, anterior-to-posterior glenohumeral joint) and is described as deep pain. Patients may also report pain at the anterior shoulder in the area of the biceps tendon. Clicking, popping, or catching in the shoulder during arm motions may be reported. However, evidence indicates that a report of clicking, catching, and popping as an individual finding likely does not differentially diagnose a labral or SLAP lesion.

There is a plethora of physical examination tools and special tests developed to diagnose labral lesions, and SLAP tears in particular. Three recent systematic reviews[2-4] presented a review of the evidence for diagnostic tests for SLAP lesions. Generally, the systematic reviews indicated that the majority of tests are not helpful for either confirming (ruling in) or screening (ruling out) SLAP lesions. The tests that have been examined in multiple studies and shown evidence to indicate that they are helpful for either confirming and/or screening SLAP lesions are the anterior slide, Yergason, compression rotation, pain provocation, anterior slide, biceps load II, and resistive supination external rotation/labral tension tests. Of particular note is the evidence for the O'Brien/active compression test. The active compression test is the most commonly investigated test for SLAP tears, and the evidence indicates that it is not recommended for use, because it is not good for either confirming or screening SLAP tears. Physical examination tests that have been examined for their diagnostic ability in only a single study and may have value but are not recommended for use until further studies are performed are the modified dynamic labral shear, biceps load I, supine flexion resistance, Kim, passive distraction, and passive compression tests. Table 10-1 summarizes the evidence for the use of physical examination tests.

Evaluation of a patient with shoulder pain who is suspected of having a SLAP tear involves the collection of patient history and performance of physical examination tests. The clinician then uses this combination of findings to arrive at a diagnosis. Several studies have examined the ability of a combination of history and physical examination tests to differentially diagnose SLAP tears. Combinations of tests that may be as helpful or more helpful than individual tests to diagnose a SLAP lesion are listed in Table 10-1. These combinations of tests seem to be better at confirming the presence of a SLAP lesion but less helpful at ruling out

Table 10-1

Summary of Evidence for Diagnosing SLAP Tears

History or Test	Confirm (Rule In)	Screen (Rule Out)
Anterior slide	√	
Yergason	√	
Compression rotation	√	
Anterior apprehension	√	√
Biceps load II	√	√
Resisted supination external rotation		
Labral tension	√	√
Pain provocation	√	√
Combinations		
History of pop, click, and catch + anterior slide	√	
Passive distraction + active compression	√	
Compression-rotation + speed + apprehension	√	

Not qualified = does not meet diagnostic thresholds. Rule in: +LR ≥ 2.0 and/or ≥ 80% specificity. Rule out: −LR ≤ 0.5 and/or ≥ 80% sensitivity.

the presence of the lesion. Clinicians should be aware that caution is warranted for the combination of tests because they were investigated in only a single study.

Recommendations for the best tests to screen and confirm the presence of a SLAP lesion are summarized in Table 10-1. The recommendations were based on a review of the evidence and the diagnostic accuracy statistics of sensitivity, specificity, positive likelihood ratio (+LR), and negative likelihood ratio (−LR). The criteria used to make recommendations were as follows: (1) the test had to be investigated by at least 2 studies and (2) the test must have a sensitivity of ≥ 80% or a +LR of ≥2.0 to recommend it for confirming the SLAP diagnosis, or a specificity of ≥ 80% and a −LR of ≤ 0.5 for screening. Recommendations for a combination of tests were based on criteria 2 only.

Conclusion

It is important that clinicians perform a comprehensive history and physical examination of a patient with a suspected SLAP lesion and not rely solely on special tests. However, when selecting which special tests to perform, clinicians should be aware of the diagnostic utility of special tests for ruling in and screening out a SLAP lesion.

References

1. Snyder SJ, Karzel RP, Del Pizzo W, Ferkel RD, Friedman MJ. SLAP lesions of the shoulder. *Arthroscopy.* 1990;6(4):274-279.
2. Dessaur WA, Magarey ME. Diagnostic accuracy of clinical tests for superior labral anterior posterior lesions: a systematic review. *J Orthop Sports Phys Ther.* 2008;38(6):341-352.
3. Hegedus EJ, Goode AP, Cook CE, et al. Which physical examination tests provide clinicians with the most value when examining the shoulder? Update of a systematic review with meta-analysis of individual tests. *Br J Sports Med.* 2012;46(14):964-978.
4. Meserve BB, Cleland JA, Boucher TR. A meta-analysis examining clinical test utilities for assessing meniscal injury. *Clin Rehabil.* 2008;22(2):143-161.

QUESTION 11

Which History and Physical Examination Diagnostic Tests Can Confirm and Screen Glenohumeral Instability?

Josie L. Harding, BS, ATC, AT and
Kellie C. Huxel Bliven, PhD, ATC

Glenohumeral (GH) instability is a common pathology in the athletic shoulder because of the joint's high degree of mobility and reliance on static and dynamic tissues, making it susceptible to injury. GH instability is classified based on either the cause or direction of the instability and is generally classified as traumatic or atraumatic. Traumatic GH instability is defined as an event that causes GH joint subluxation or a frank dislocation and is either spontaneously reduced or requires reduction.[1] Atraumatic instability is the most common event and is the result of generalized ligamentous laxity or is secondary to repetitive overhead motion.

GH instability is also categorized based on the direction of the instability: anterior, posterior, inferior, or multidirectional. Anterior instability is the most common direction, occurring in about 95% of instability cases.[1] It is frequently caused by repetitive microtrauma involving external rotation when the GH joint is abducted to 90 degrees. Anterior instability commonly manifests as muscle weakness of the rotator cuff and long head of the biceps.[1] Posterior instability is caused by repetitive microtrauma involving longitudinal forces across the humerus, through

Huxel Bliven KC, ed. *Quick Questions in the Shoulder: Expert Advice in Sports Medicine* (pp 59-62).

internal rotation with the GH at 90 degrees and horizontal adduction. Posterior instability is commonly associated with nonspecific, chronic shoulder pain. This instability accounts for only 2% to 5% of all cases.[1,2] Inferior instability typically does not occur in isolation; it is commonly involved with multidirectional instability (MDI). MDI is a result of repetitive microtrauma imposed on a congenitally lax and redundant joint capsule. Patients with MDI often present with a variety of symptoms that range from vague shoulder pain without perception of instability to daily occurrences of subluxations or dislocations with activities of daily living. Typically, patients have reduced muscular strength, scapula upward rotation, and decreased neuromuscular control of shoulder function.[1]

As with any injury, diagnosis via an accurate and thorough examination is the key to managing a patient with GH instability. It is essential to gain an appropriate history and mechanism of injury, as well as the level of external trauma applied at the onset of the injury. History obtained from the patient should involve chief complaint, age, arm dominance, and sport. Although most cases of GH instability involve vague symptoms, common complaints will include pain, popping, catching, locking, an unstable sensation, stiffness, and swelling. When pain is reported, it is important to ask about the location and quality of the pain and any aggravating and relieving factors. It is also essential to determine when the symptoms first started occurring, the frequency of symptoms, and positions or activities that result in the instability episodes.[1]

Clinicians should use a systematic approach to evaluating a patient who is suspected to have GH instability. Kuhn et al[3] developed an approach that focuses on obtaining information about frequency, etiology, direction, and severity (FEDS) that aims to help classify GH instability and is based on answers to the following 5 questions: (1) Confirm dislocation: Did your shoulder slip or fall out? Is it loose? (2) Frequency: Has the instability occurred one time (isolated), 2 to 5 times in a year (occasional), or more than 5 times in a year (frequent)? (3) Etiology: Did the instability occur as a result of trauma, or was it atraumatic? (4) Direction: Did your shoulder go out in front (anterior), out the bottom (inferior), or out the back (posterior)? (5) Severity: Did you need help to get your shoulder back in (dislocation/subluxation)?[3] Responses to these questions should assist the clinician in classifying the instability, which can then be followed up with a clinical examination to confirm the diagnosis.

There are several physical examination and special tests designed to detect GH instability. The use of just one special test is not recommended for making a diagnosis; instead, a combination of special tests should be used to improve the accuracy of diagnoses. In a systematic review by Hegedus et al,[4] a series of clinical tests were recommended for anterior instability because of their specificities, sensitivities, and likelihood ratios. The apprehension, relocation, and surprise tests,

Table 11-1

Special Tests for Posterior Instability

Combination Clinical Test	Confirm (Rule In)	Screen (Rule Out)
Apprehension, relocation, and surprise	√	√
Kim and jerk		√

Table 11-2

Special Tests and Diagnostic Values for Anterior Instability

Clinical Test	Confirm (Rule In)	Screen (Rule Out)	Specificity	Sensitivity	Likelihood Ratio
Apprehension	√				17.2 (strongest positive)
Relocation	√		90%		
Surprise		√		82%	0.25 (negative)
Posterior apprehension	√		95%		
Jerk	√		98%	73%	

when used in combination, have the best clinical utility to rule in or out anterior instability (Table 11-1). Specifically apprehension and relocation offer the best specificity (98%) and sensitivity (81%). Apprehension alone has the strongest positive likelihood ratio (17.2), making it a good test to rule in anterior instability. The surprise test presented with the strongest sensitivity (82%) and negative likelihood ratio (0.25), making it a good test for ruling out anterior instability (Table 11-2).[4]

Common tests for clinically assessing posterior instability are the load and shift, jerk, Kim, and posterior apprehension tests (see Table 11-2). Posterior apprehension has a strong specificity (95%) and a sensitivity of only 58%, meaning a positive test will rule in posterior instability.[4] The Kim and jerk tests, when used together, have a good diagnostic accuracy in ruling out instability and a negative test sensitivity (97%).[2] The jerk test alone has a 98% specificity and a 73% sensitivity.[5]

The sulcus sign and hyperabduction tests are the most commonly used tests in the clinical setting to assess multidirectional instability. Both of these tests will primarily assess inferior instability by putting the inferior GH ligament on stress. There is currently no diagnostic accuracy reported for these tests, but they stress the inferior GH ligament.[5] This ligament is a primary static stabilizer in the GH joint, which means any disruption to this ligament can cause multidirectional instability.

When approaching a patient with suspected GH instability, it would be beneficial for the clinician to apply the FEDS system to help direct the physical examination. Once the clinician obtains appropriate information from the FEDS system to properly classify the type of instability, he or she can direct his or her physical examination by applying the recommended tests to rule in or out the GH instability suspected. The apprehension, relocation, and surprise tests, when used in combination, have a strong specificity, making them the most reliable tests for ruling in (confirming) anterior instability. The Kim and jerk tests, when used together, are recommended to use when ruling out (screening) posterior instability. Tests used to assess multidirectional instability include the sulcus and hyperabduction tests, but their diagnostic accuracy values have not been reported.

References

1. Finnoff JT, Doucette S, Hicken G. Glenohumeral instability and dislocation. *Phys Med Rehabil Clin N Am.* 2004;15(3):v-vi, 575-605.
2. Provencher MT, LeClere LE, King S, et al. Posterior instability of the shoulder: diagnosis and management. *Am J Sports Med.* 2011;39(4):874-886.
3. Kuhn JE, Helmer TT, Dunn WR, Throckmorton VT. Development and reliability testing of the frequency, etiology, direction, and severity (FEDS) system for classifying glenohumeral instability. *J Shoulder Elbow Surg.* 2011;20(4):548-556.
4. Hegedus EJ, Goode AP, Cook CE, et al. Which physical examination tests provide clinicians with the most value when examining the shoulder? Update of a systematic review with meta-analysis of individual tests. *Br J Sports Med.* 2012;46(14):964-978.
5. Sciascia AD, Spigelman T, Kibler WB, Uhl TL. Frequency of use of clinical shoulder examination tests by experienced shoulder surgeons. *J Athl Train.* 2012;47(4):457-466.

QUESTION 12

Which Clinical and Diagnostic Imaging Tests Are Most Effective for Diagnosing Rotator Cuff Disease?

Matthew K. Walsworth, MD, PT and
Lori A. Michener, PhD, PT, ATC, SCS

Rotator cuff disease (RCD) is a spectrum of pathology involving tendinopathy, partial-thickness tearing, or full-thickness tearing of one or more of the 4 rotator cuff tendons in isolation or in conjunction with bursitis of the subacromial bursa (Figures 12-1 and 12-2). The most frequent cause of shoulder pain and the most frequently encountered category of RCD is subacromial impingement syndrome (SIS).[1,2] SIS is likely multifactorial in etiology, and causative theories have been the subject of controversy. The extrinsic theory of SIS attributes the cause to direct tendon/bursa compression by acromial morphology, glenohumeral capsular laxity or tightness, and altered scapulohumeral mechanics. The intrinsic theory of SIS favors tendon overload and overuse. It is likely that elements of both theories are at play, but it is unclear whether one is predominant. Regardless of etiology, the presentation of SIS can involve bursitis, tendinopathy, and partial- or full-thickness tendon tear.[1-3]

The differential diagnosis for suspected RCD is broad and includes internal derangements such as labral lesions, instability, acromioclavicular joint pathology,

Huxel Bliven KC, ed. *Quick Questions in the Shoulder: Expert Advice in Sports Medicine* (pp 63-67).

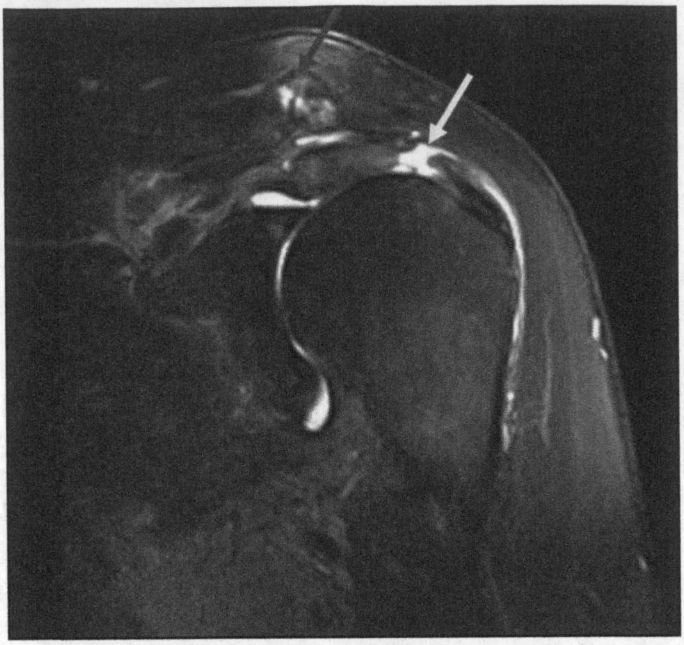

Figure 12-1. Coronal short tau inversion recovery (STIR) MRI demonstrating a full-thickness supraspinatus tear (white arrow) in addition to degenerative changes of the acromioclavicular joint (dark arrow).

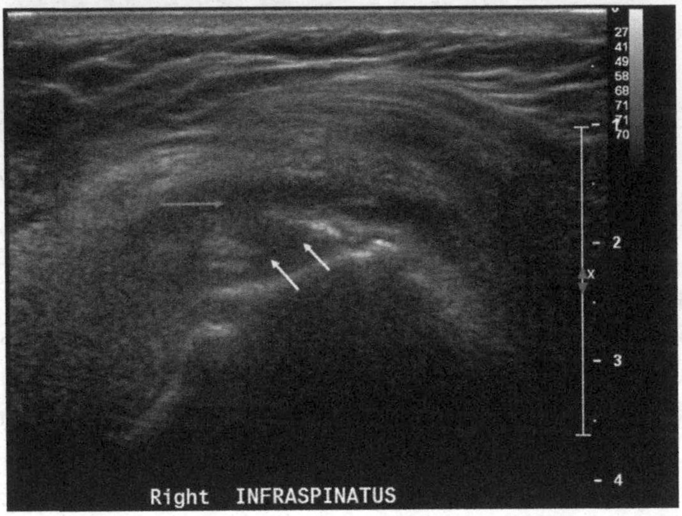

Figure 12-2. Long axis ultrasound image of the infraspinatus depicting a full-thickness tear of the tendon (white arrows) and fluid and debris within the subacromial/subdeltoid bursa (dark arrow).

adhesive capsulitis, neuropathies about the shoulder region, and cervical radiculopathy. The first steps toward diagnosis are obtaining the patient's history and examining him or her. With RCD, most of the patient history is nonspecific for confirming the diagnosis. Younger athletes may describe traumatic rotator cuff injury related to throwing or contact injury. Although most patients with RCD complain of pain, it is nonspecific. The location of pain in RCD is most commonly in the subacromial region but may also be in the mid-humerus, scapular spine, and midclavicular regions. Although nonspecific, history findings that increase the probability of full-thickness rotator cuff tear include age greater than 65 years and night pain. However, this is less applicable in a young, athletic population. Weakness, stiffness, loss of motion, pain with overhead activities, and crepitus are also common but nonspecific.[1-4]

Clinical tests for RCD may be divided into those that test the function of the rotator cuff musculotendinous structures and those that are pain provocation tests for SIS.[1,2] A daunting number of clinical tests are purported to be useful to diagnose RCD. However, some of these tests have not been investigated adequately, and some others have demonstrated poor diagnostic accuracy. To best use and interpret test results, it is important to have an understanding of diagnostic accuracy statistics, such as sensitivity, specificity, and likelihood ratios. Based on the current best evidence, the recommended clinical tests to evaluate for SIS and RCD are listed in Table 12-1.[1,2,4]

Historically, the gold standard for diagnosing RCD has been surgery. However, because many patients with RCD do not require surgery and because imaging is frequently used in clinical decision making, magnetic resonance imaging (MRI) or ultrasound (US) often serves as a practical reference standard for diagnosis. Valuable information that can be obtained from imaging includes an assessment of the location and severity of the tendinopathy or tear. Other factors that are also apparent on imaging and may aid in decision making include degree of retraction of the torn tendon, atrophy, and fatty infiltration of the torn musculotendinous unit. MR arthrography or conventional MRI in particular can also demonstrate other derangements such as labral pathology.[3,5]

The choice of imaging modality for RCD depends on a variety of factors, including the suspected clinical diagnosis, availability of various imaging modalities, and patient and clinician preferences. The initial imaging evaluation frequently begins with radiographs. Radiographs are of limited utility in RCD, but they may demonstrate abnormalities helpful in narrowing the differential diagnosis, such as acromion morphologic abnormalities suggestive of extrinsic impingement, superior migration of the humeral head (which can be seen in full-thickness RCD), acromioclavicular degenerative disease, or osseous abnormalities associated with instability. MR arthrography has demonstrated superior diagnostic accuracy over all other imaging modalities. However, MR arthrography requires a minimally invasive procedure in which a radiologist injects gadolinium contrast into the glenohumeral joint under fluoroscopic guidance before performance of an MRI. This procedure incurs a small degree of risk and expense compared with conventional MRI. The accuracy of MR arthrography in the diagnosis of RCD is closely followed by that of conventional MRI and US. However, MR arthrography and conventional MRI offer advantages over US in diagnosing other shoulder lesions, such as labral pathology. Furthermore, US imaging of the rotator cuff is operator dependent and generally less available in the United States.[5]

Table 12-1

Evidence-Based Clinical Tests for Rotator Cuff Disease

Test	SIS/Tendinopathy/ Partial-Thickness RCD		Full-Thickness RCD	
	Rule In	*Rule Out*	*Rule In*	*Rule Out*
Painful arc	X	X	X	
Full can (pain or weakness)	X	X		X
Drop arm	X	X	X	
Resisted external rotation (pain or weakness; marked weakness criteria for full-thickness tears)	X	X	X	X
Empty can		X		X
Neer		X		
Hawkins-Kennedy		X		
External rotation lag sign			X	
Internal rotation lag/lift-off test			X	X
Belly press			X	
Infraspinatus atrophy			X	
Combinations				
Hawkins-Kennedy, painful arc, external rotation	3+/3	3−/5		
Hawkins-Kennedy, Neer, painful arc, empty can, external rotation	≥3+/5	≤3+/5		
Drop arm, painful arc, resisted external rotation			3+/3	3−/3

References

1. Alqunaee M, Galvin R, Fahey T. Diagnostic accuracy of clinical tests for subacromial impingement syndrome: a systematic review and meta-analysis. *Arch Phys Med Rehabil.* 2012;93(2):229-236.
2. Hermans J, Luime JJ, Meuffels DE, Reijman M, Simel DL, Bierma-Zeinstra SM. Does this patient with shoulder pain have rotator cuff disease? The Rational Clinical Examination systematic review. *JAMA.* 2013;310(8):837-847.
3. Morag Y, Jacobson JA, Miller B, De Maeseneer M, Girish G, Jamadar D. MR imaging of rotator cuff injury: what the clinician needs to know. *Radiographics.* 2006;26(4):1045-1065.
4. Hegedus EJ, Goode AP, Cook CE, et al. Which physical examination tests provide clinicians with the most value when examining the shoulder? Update of a systematic review with meta-analysis of individual tests. *Br J Sports Med.* 2012;46(14):964-978.

5. de Jesus JO, Parker L, Frangos AJ, Nazarian LN. Accuracy of MRI, MR arthrography, and ultrasound in the diagnosis of rotator cuff tears: a meta-analysis. *AJR Am J Roentgenol.* 2009;192(6):1701-1707.

QUESTION 13

WHAT CONSTITUTES A HIGH-QUALITY, EFFECTIVE CLINICAL ASSESSMENT OF THORACIC OUTLET SYNDROME?

Gail P. Parr, PhD, ATC

Clinicians have long been frustrated in their efforts to diagnose and treat thoracic outlet syndrome (TOS). Varying views on the definition, etiology, signs, and symptoms of TOS have resulted in controversies that continue to influence the implementation of assessment techniques. The lack of evidenced-based best practice presents challenges for clinicians in their efforts to diagnose and manage TOS effectively.

TOS is a condition that produces upper extremity symptoms resulting from compression of a neurovascular bundle at the thoracic outlet. Three sites of compression include the cervical rib and the scalene musculature, beneath the clavicle in the costoclavicular space, and the subcoracoid space.

TOS includes 3 classifications reflecting the structures being compressed: neurogenic TOS (NTOS), involving compression of the brachial plexus; arterial TOS (ATOS), compression of the subclavian artery; and venous TOS (VTOS), compression of the subclavian vein. NTOS can be either true NTOS (tNTOS) or disputed NTOS (dNTOS). tNTOS is associated with objective findings of weakness

Huxel Bliven KC, ed. *Quick Questions in the Shoulder: Expert Advice in Sports Medicine* (pp 69-73).

and/or sensory deficit; dNTOS involves weakness and/or sensory deficit based on subjective information and not confirmed with objective testing.[1]

Although the incidence of TOS is difficult to measure, research suggests that NTOS ranks highest, comprising 95% to 98% of cases, while vascular forms of TOS account for 3% to 5% of incidents.[2] The majority of TOS cases involve individuals aged 20 to 50 years. TOS is seldom seen in adolescents and rarely in children. The incidence of TOS is higher among females, with an estimated female-to-male ratio of 3:1.[2]

TOS has been attributed to several etiological factors. Congenital anomalies can affect bony and soft tissue structures. Bony pathology includes anomalies of the cervical rib, an elongated transverse process of the seventh cervical vertebra, and an enlarged scalene tubercle. Soft tissue anomalies include enlarged scalene muscles, pectoralis minor muscles, and costoclavicular ligaments. Etiological factors can also include trauma involving the neck or shoulder.[3] Bone remodeling subsequent to a fracture of the clavicle or first rib can result in bony lesions. Muscle hypertrophy, excessive muscle contraction, and muscle spasm can develop after trauma. Postural and repetitive occupational movements have also been identified as potential causes of TOS. Ergonomically inappropriate computer stations can subject an individual to repetitive adverse stress to the neck and arms. Poor posture can increase susceptibility to TOS as a result of the size and shape of the thoracic outlet changing over time. Dysfunction or imbalances of the muscles that govern the neck and shoulder can also be predisposing factors.[2]

In general, TOS is characterized by pain, paresthesia, weakness, and discomfort in the upper limb. The types of TOS present with varying clinical features, depending on the structure being compressed. Symptoms can be unilateral or bilateral and can include both neurogenic and vascular components. It is important for clinicians to appreciate that the presentation of signs and symptoms can vary significantly among individuals diagnosed with TOS. Table 13-1 summarizes common clinical features of the classifications of TOS.

Clinical diagnosis of TOS requires a detailed history and examination. It is important to understand that any number of the signs and symptoms are associated with other conditions involving the head, neck, shoulder, and upper extremity. As such, it becomes essential for clinicians to differentiate TOS from other conditions that may be present or exist in addition to TOS. Because TOS is sustained by a relatively small number of individuals, it can be inadvertently overlooked by the clinician in favor of a more common condition.

Obtaining a detailed and comprehensive history is an integral component of any clinical assessment. It is particularly valuable when TOS is suspected. The significance of the history is attributed to the absence of provocative tests that have the sensitivity and specificity to confirm TOS.[4] The history should include not only

Table 13-1

Clinical Signs and Symptoms of Thoracic Outlet Syndrome

ATOS	VTOS
• Spontaneous; following intense arm activity • Pain in hand and fingers • Claudication • Absent or decreased arterial pulse • Digital ischemia that yields paresthesia, coldness, and pallor • Shoulder and neck pain uncommon • Typically unilateral	• Spontaneous; following intense arm activity • Edema of the arm • Pain may or may not be present • Feeling of stiffness or heaviness in upper arm • Paresthesia in fingers and hand • Cyanosis • Venous engorgement • Neck pain uncommon • Typically unilateral
tNTOS	**dNTOS**
• History of neck trauma before symptoms • Trauma, often car accident or repetitive stress • Pain, paresthesia, numbness in the arm and hand (medial or lateral, depending on upper or lower plexus involvement) • Cold intolerance • Overactive sympathetic nervous system resulting in cold intolerance, hand coldness, and color changes • Hand weakness; loss of dexterity • Atrophy of thenar or hypothenar eminence • Anterior neck pain • Typically unilateral • Confirmed through neurological testing	• History of neck trauma before symptoms • Trauma, often car accident or repetitive stress • Pain in forearm, wrist, and hand • Pain at rest and at night • Paresthesia in fingers, typically nocturnal, that awakens patient • Cold intolerance • Overactive sympathetic nervous system resulting in cold intolerance, hand coldness, and color changes • Hand weakness; loss of dexterity • Neck and shoulder pain • Neurological testing is normal

Adapted from Watson LA, Pizzari T, Balster S. Thoracic outlet syndrome part 2: conservative management of thoracic outlet. *Man Ther.* 2010;15(4):305-314 and
Nichols AW. Diagnosis and management of thoracic outlet syndrome. *Curr Sports Med Rep.* 2009;8(5):240-249 and
Hooper TL, Denton J, McGalliard MK, Brismee JM, Sizer PS Jr. Thoracic outlet syndrome: a controversial clinical condition. Part 1: anatomy, and clinical examination/diagnosis. *J Man Manip Ther.* 2010;18(2):74-83.

current symptoms but also information from before the onset of symptoms. Given the etiology of TOS, noting any previous trauma to the neck and shoulder can provide important information. Similarly, questions concerning the performance of activities that involve repetitive stress are also noteworthy. For both tNTOS and dNTOS, a common finding is symptoms that developed after an automobile accident or subsequent to repetitive stresses associated with daily work.[5] Understanding the onset of symptoms is also essential. A finding that symptoms occur throughout the day as compared with awakening an individual during the night is valuable in the overall assessment. Clinicians should ask questions regarding the location, nature, severity, frequency, and duration of pain or other unusual sensations (eg, paresthesia, numbness, tingling).

The physical examination should begin with a postural assessment. Focus should be the upper body, including position of the head, shoulders, cervical spine, thoracic spine, scapulae, and arms. The presence of kyphosis, forward head, posterior tilt, downward rotation, and/or depression of the scapulae is particularly noteworthy because each can contribute to increased loading of the brachial plexus.[5]

The examination should continue with a visual inspection of the upper extremities. The presence of atypical skin color, edema, or muscle atrophy (particularly of the thenar and hypothenar eminence muscles) should be noted. Cyanosis or paleness can be indicative of vascular compression, whereas atrophy suggests nerve involvement. Arm swelling and distended veins at the shoulder and chest wall are associated exclusively with VTOS. In comparison, color changes and ischemia suggest ATOS.

Palpation can also elicit relevant information. The supraclavicular fossa should be palpated for pain because the brachial plexus is located in that area. The hands should be palpated for temperature because coldness can be indicative of ATOS. Palpation can also be used to assess cutaneous sensation and pulse.

The physical examination should proceed to assessment of active and passive range of motion (ROM) of the cervical spine, shoulder, elbow, wrist, and fingers. Scapulothoracic motion should also be evaluated. The ROM component should determine the presence of deficiencies, abnormal movements, or reproduction of symptoms. Manual muscle testing can also be used to assess any weakness.

A neurological examination is an essential component of the physical examination. The results of motor, sensory, and deep tendon reflex testing can provide information that indicates the potential for NTOS.

Provocative tests are typically an integral part of a clinical assessment. Historically, several tests (eg, Adson maneuver, Allen test, Roos stress test, Wright test) have been used to confirm the diagnosis of TOS. However, recent research, along with the absence of quality, evidence-based research, challenges the reliability, sensitivity, and specificity of these tests. It has been reported that provocative tests for TOS have a low sensitivity, with an average rate of 72%, and a low specificity, with an average of 53%.[6] It has also been reported that provocative tests for TOS are associated with high rates of false-positive findings.[7] Accordingly, these tests are not considered reliable. It is important for clinicians to recognize the limitations of provocative tests in assessing TOS.

Clinicians must understand that there is no single test or framework for diagnosing TOS. Clinicians are challenged with recognizing that signs and symptoms common to TOS are associated with several other conditions (eg, carpal tunnel syndrome [CTS], complex regional pain syndrome, Raynaud phenomenon, and brachial plexus trauma). The more familiar clinicians are with TOS and other conditions involving the upper extremities, shoulder complex, and cervical and thoracic spines, the better positioned they will be to perform effective assessments. As previously mentioned, a detailed and comprehensive history can provide key information. For example, determining the location and path/direction of pain or other unusual sensations can help clinicians differentiate between a symptom of CTS and a symptom of NTOS. In CTS, the symptoms typically originate in the hand and move up the forearm; the symptoms associated with NTOS radiate from the neck and travel toward the hand.[1] Clinicians must take a position that permits differential diagnosis rather than an isolated diagnosis.

Based on their findings, clinicians should be prepared to consult with a physician. A high-quality clinical assessment can provide physicians with information that will guide the further assessment and management of the condition.

References

1. Christo PJ, McGreevy K. Updated perspectives on neurogenic thoracic outlet syndrome. *Curr Pain Headache Rep.* 2011;15(1):14-21.
2. Watson LA, Pizzari T, Balster S. Thoracic outlet syndrome part 2: conservative management of thoracic outlet. *Man Ther.* 2010;15(4):305-314.
3. Davidovic LB, Kostic DM, Jakovljevic NS, Kuzmanovic IL, Simic TM. Vascular thoracic outlet syndrome. *World J Surg.* 2003;27(5):545-550.
4. Nichols AW. Diagnosis and management of thoracic outlet syndrome. *Curr Sports Med Rep.* 2009;8(5):240-249.
5. Hooper TL, Denton J, McGalliard MK, Brismee JM, Sizer PS Jr. Thoracic outlet syndrome: a controversial clinical condition. Part 1: anatomy, and clinical examination/diagnosis. *J Man Manip Ther.* 2010;18(2):74-83.
6. Nord KM, Kapoor P, Fisher J, et al. False positive rate of thoracic outlet syndrome diagnostic maneuvers. *Electromyogr Clin Neurophysiol.* 2008;48(2):67-74.
7. Cook C, Hegedus EJ. *Orthopedic Physical Examination Tests: An Evidence-Based Approach.* Upper Saddle River, NJ: Pearson Prentice Hall; 2008.

QUESTION 14

What Is Effort Thrombosis, and How Is It Diagnosed and Treated?

Matthew K. Walsworth, MD, PT and Jonathan K. Park, MD

Effort thrombosis, also known as Paget-Schroetter syndrome, is an uncommon but important entity in the athletic population. It is important because, if not diagnosed and treated early, it can result in chronic disability and, in some cases (up to 20%), life-threatening pulmonary embolism.[1-3] It is a subtype of thoracic outlet syndrome (TOS) involving deep vein thrombosis (DVT) of the subclavian and/or axillary vein. Although it classically occurs in the dominant arm of throwing athletes, there are many reported cases involving nonthrowing athletes as well as manual laborers. The reported incidence in the general population is believed to be 1 to 2 per 100,000, but this may be an underestimate because many consider this entity underdiagnosed. The incidence among athletes is likely higher than that of the general population.[1]

The broader entity of TOS is somewhat controversial. TOS involves compression of one or more neurovascular structures of the brachial plexus, subclavian artery, and/or subclavian vein as they traverse the space between the clavicle and first rib.

Huxel Bliven KC, ed. *Quick Questions in the Shoulder: Expert Advice in Sports Medicine* (pp 75-79).

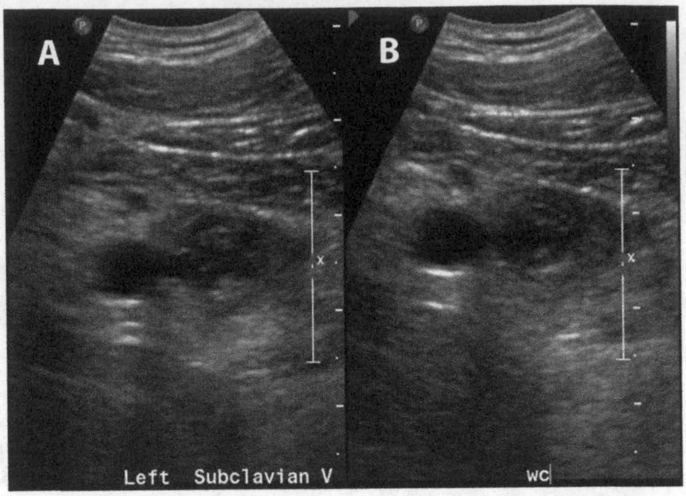

Figure 14-1. (A) Grayscale ultrasound imaging depicting the subclavian artery and vein with echogenic thrombus in the subclavian vein prior to manual compression. (B) With manual compression using the ultrasound probe, the vein is not compressible, confirming the presence of thrombus.

The neurologic form (brachial plexus compression) of TOS is considered the most common,[1] but the diagnostic criteria and true incidence of this form are highly controversial.[4] The second most common form of TOS affects the subclavian and/or axillary veins in the region of the costoclavicular junction. Effort thrombosis falls into this category. The 3 subtypes of venous TOS follow: (1) effort thrombosis (the focus of this chapter); (2) iatrogenic thrombosis, related to devices such as catheters and pacemakers; and (3) intermittent/positional venous compression. The diagnosis of effort thrombosis is far less controversial than that of the neurologic or arterial types of TOS because clinical signs and symptoms can be confirmed with imaging evidence of venous thrombosis (Figure 14-1). In further distinction, there are separate anatomic spaces for potential compression of the subclavian vein as compared with the subclavian artery and brachial plexus as they traverse the thoracic outlet. Specifically, the vein is contained in a more anterior space than the artery and brachial plexus. The space containing the subclavian vein is bordered by the scalenus anticus muscle posteriorly, the subclavius muscle anteriorly, the first rib inferiorly, and the clavicle superiorly.[1,2,4] Vein compression within this space can occur by the combination of decreased space and repetitive shoulder activity. Factors that decrease the space include muscle hypertrophy of the scalene, subclavius, or pectoralis minor and soft tissue and osseous abnormalities such as anomalous fibrous bands and posttraumatic deformity of the clavicle. Repetitive venous compression is thought to occur particularly as a result of repetitive abduction and external rotation, particularly in throwers. This results in repetitive microtrauma that theoretically causes a chronic local inflammatory process, which subsequently forms fibrotic tissue around the vein, which decreases the mobility of the vein. The venous hypomobility leads to thrombosis formation caused by repetitive stretching,

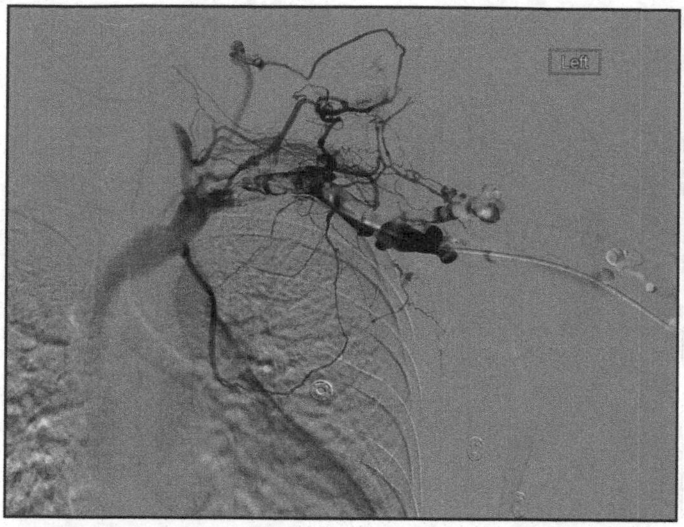

Figure 14-2. Venogram depicting near-occlusive thrombus in the axillary and subclavian veins of the left upper extremity. Note that the more central veins are filling largely via collateral veins.

microtearing, and/or compression of the vein. Alternatively, thrombosis may be initiated by single compressive events in sports such as wrestling.[1-3]

The classic presentation of a patient with effort thrombosis includes a painful, swollen, discolored (bluish) arm. Patients frequently describe the arm as "heavy." They may have visually appreciable dilated superficial veins in the arm, chest wall, and neck. Patients are typically symptomatic within 24 hours after an inciting event.[1-3,5] Physical examination should include assessment of the arterial and neurologic status in the involved limb because the differential diagnosis includes the neurologic and arterial forms of TOS, cervical radiculopathy, brachial plexopathy, and a variety of neuropathies that may affect the shoulder region. Although rare in the young athletic population, malignant processes should be considered because they may lead to thrombus formation caused by a resultant hypercoagulable state or compression of the neurovascular structures in the thoracic outlet region.[2,5] Traditional clinical tests for TOS (eg, Adson test, Wright test) are not helpful in diagnosing effort thrombosis because they are more pertinent to the neurologic or arterial subtypes, although they are of debatable diagnostic accuracy for even those forms of TOS.[2,4]

Although conventional venography is the historical gold standard for diagnosis (Figure 14-2), duplex ultrasonography is the initial recommended imaging modality to evaluate for DVT because it is accurate (sensitivity 78% to 100%, specificity 82% to 100%), noninvasive, and relatively inexpensive and does not involve ionizing radiation. However, the subclavian and other central veins can not always be adequately visualized with ultrasound. Therefore, nondiagnostic or false-negative ultrasound studies may occur. In these cases, magnetic resonance venography, computed tomography venography, or conventional venography may be needed for further evaluation. In cases in which the diagnosis is made after ultrasound,

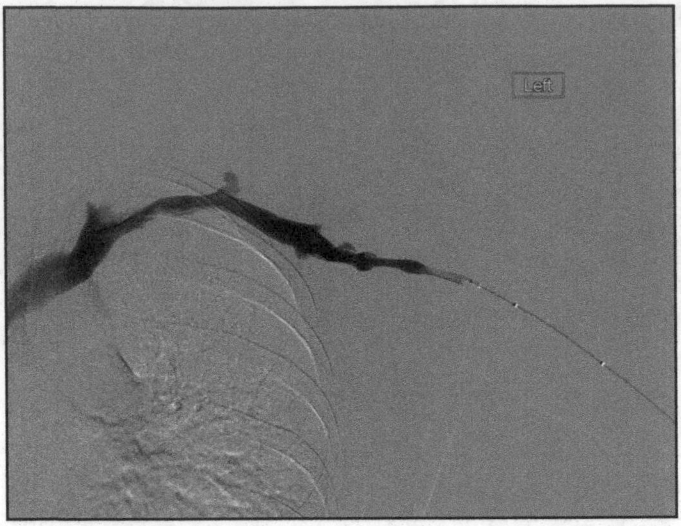

Figure 14-3. Venogram depicting markedly improved patency of the left axillary and subclavian veins of the left upper extremity after thrombolysis and angioplasty. Extensive filling of the collateral veins is no longer seen. There is a small residual peripheral filling defect in the left subclavian vein, which may represent mild refractory thrombus or a region of refractory stenosis.

chest radiography may be useful to evaluate for osseous abnormalities and apical lung masses.[1-3,5] Although the presence of cervical ribs has been implicated in the forms of TOS that affect the brachial plexus and subclavian artery, these relatively posterior structures are unlikely to cause venous forms of TOS such as effort thrombosis.[1,2]

When clinical findings are strongly suggestive of effort thrombosis (particularly if imaging findings are confirmatory), conventional venography should be pursued without delay because initial management with catheter-directed endovascular interventions can be performed at the same time. Typically, the initial management of effort thrombosis involves catheter-directed thrombolysis using tissue plasminogen activator, sometimes in combination with thrombectomy devices and/or balloon angioplasty (Figure 14-3). Thrombolysis is most effective when performed early, with chances for success diminishing as days and weeks pass. Although it is generally agreed upon that initial thrombolysis is critical, some controversy exists as to the optimal management once venous patency has been restored. Although prospective trials are lacking, most evidence suggests that definitive management with early surgical decompression is usually necessary to prevent recurrent thrombotic episodes.[1-3,5] Medical management with anticoagulation therapy alone has generally yielded higher recurrence rates, greater disability, and increased risk of life-threatening pulmonary embolism than has surgery.[1-3,5] Even so, some authors suggest a trial of anticoagulation and physical therapy focused on stretching the potentially implicated soft tissue structures because this may be appropriate for some patients because of the risks associated with surgery.[3] Patient preferences, goals, and expectations should be considered when choosing the management strategy. Regardless of the management strategy used, 3 to 6 months of anticoagulation therapy with repeat imaging is generally recommended.[1-3,5]

References

1. Illig KA, Doyle AJ. A comprehensive review of Paget-Schroetter syndrome. *J Vasc Surg.* 2010;51(6):1538-1547.
2. Mall NA, Van Thiel GS, Heard WM, Paletta GA, Bush-Joseph C, Bach BR Jr. Paget-Schroetter syndrome: a review of effort thrombosis of the upper extremity from a sports medicine perspective. *Sports Health.* 2013;5(4):353-356.
3. Thompson RW. Comprehensive management of subclavian vein effort thrombosis. *Semin Intervent Radiol.* 2012;29(1):44-51.
4. Hooper TL, Denton J, McGalliard MK, Brismee JM, Sizer PS Jr. Thoracic outlet syndrome: a controversial clinical condition. Part 1: anatomy, and clinical examination/diagnosis. *J Man Manip Ther.* 2010;18(2):74-83.
5. Joffe HV, Goldhaber SZ. Upper-extremity deep vein thrombosis. *Circulation.* 2002;106(14): 1874-1880.

QUESTION 15

What Are Common Causes of Cervical Radiculopathy, and What Clinical Tests Can Be Used to Diagnose It?

Lee N. Marinko, PT, ScD, OCS, FAAOMPT

It is important that clinicians be able to identify and differentiate sources of shoulder and neck pain in athletes. Neck pain and injuries are common in the athletic population, with most being benign in nature and the result of minor sprains, strains, or contusions. Athletes who perform repetitive overhead motion or are engaged in competition that involves contact are more likely than others to report an episode of neck pain in their lifetime. Cervical radiculopathy is a type of neck pain defined as radiating pain in the upper limb, usually experienced in a pattern consistent with a specific spinal nerve distribution.[1] This pain complaint can present in a manner similar to that of the pain associated with muscle or joint injuries yet can result in disruption of neuromuscular function and impaired performance. An understanding of its common causes and a comprehensive clinical examination are critical to identify spinal nerve involvement and initiate intervention accordingly.

Huxel Bliven KC, ed. *Quick Questions in the Shoulder: Expert Advice in Sports Medicine* (pp 81-85).

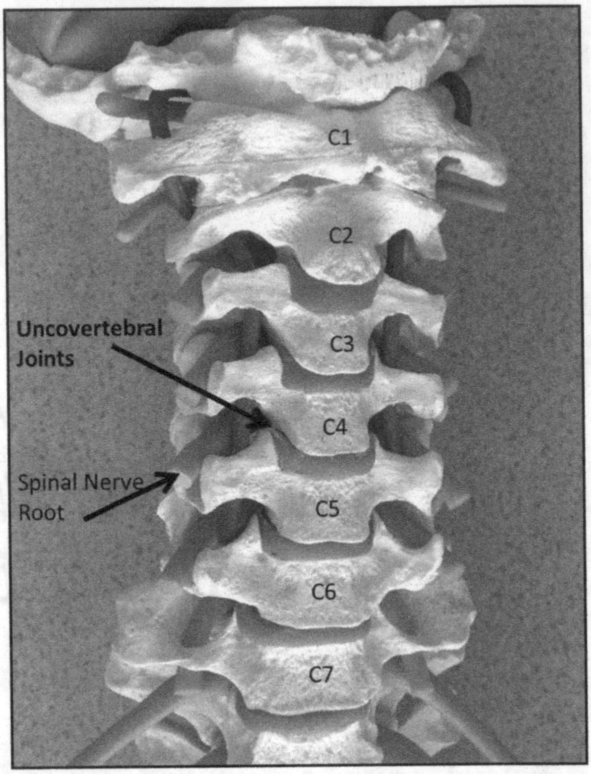

Figure 15-1. Uncovertebral joints.

Cervical radiculopathy can be caused by compression or irritation of the spinal nerve segments as they are exiting the lateral intervertebral foramen.[1] There are a number of factors that may result in irritation and potential compression and must be considered when an athlete presents with this pain. First, the cervical vertebrae are the smallest yet most mobile of the vertebral joints in the spinal column. The typical vertebrae between C3 and C7 have small, curved bodies with raised lateral hooks called uncovertebral joints (Figure 15-1). These joints articulate with the adjacent vertebral body, so each spinal segment consists of the superior vertebral body, the intervertebral disk, and the inferior vertebral body. In the normal healthy intervertebral disk, the space between each spinal segment is maintained, and the disk helps to reduce the loading on the small uncovertebral joints. This role is important because these small synovium-lined joints are not designed to sustain large amounts of forces in function. Degeneration and thinning of the intervertebral disk result in increased compression forces through the uncovertebral joints, which can result in inflammatory processes and degenerative changes. These changes over time can lead to reduced space in the intervertebral foramen and compression on the exiting spinal nerve root.

Another way the spinal nerve root can become compressed is with repetitive movement and/or sustained postures. Maintaining stability of the head and neck during upper extremity movements is the role of the deep stabilizing muscles of the spine. Active contraction of the anterior muscles (longus colli and capitis) is essential to offset the large extensive forces produced by the trapezii that are working to facilitate upward rotation of the scapula in reaching tasks.[2] In research associated with chronic neck pain, these anterior muscles have been shown to be diminished in their action. Interventions that emphasize activation can significantly reduce pain and disability. Altered stability by the anterior muscles can lead to excessive stresses to the intervertebral disc and articulating joints, thereby leading to inflammation and degeneration, again resulting in decreased foraminal space and spinal nerve compression.

Movement of the cervical spine also has an effect on the size of the intervertebral foramen and in the cervical spine and can have a direct impact on compression of the spinal nerves. Movement in all vertebral joints is coupled, so that motion in any one plane results in an automatic and often imperceptible movement in another plane. This coupled motion in the cervical spine will directly affect the shape and size of the intervertebral foramen. Specifically, lateral flexion or side-bending of the neck results in the cervical vertebra moving laterally and rotating to the same side, causing closure of the same-side foramen. Rotation results in closure on the same-side foramen, and extension of the cervical spine can reduce the size of the foramen by up to 20% in healthy adults.[3] Sustaining any of these positions alone or in combination over time may result in excessive compressive and shearing forces to the joints and the intervertebral disc as well as the sensitive spinal nerves, resulting in inflammation and radicular symptoms.

Examination for cervical radiculopathy can be fairly simple, with a combination of clear patient history and selecting the appropriate clinical tests. A cluster of positive examination findings has been found to increase the likelihood of diagnostic accuracy for cervical radiculopathy. The 4 tests that have been described are Spurling's test, the distraction test, the upper limb tension test, and involved cervical rotation less than 60 degrees. Spurling's test has been described as a moderately specific test, meaning that when performed accurately, a positive result is indicative of a true spinal nerve compression (Figure 15-2).[4] The test is performed with the patient in a seated position, and his or her head is moved into a combination of extension, side-bending, and rotation to the side of the pain. If this movement reproduces or increases the individual's pain, the result is positive. If the procedure is painful, a follow-up test is to apply a distraction force through the head and neck in the end position. If during distraction the pain goes away, that is considered confirmation that the pain is the result of compression to the spinal nerve. If no pain is produced in this position, an axial compressive load through the spine can be applied. The distraction test is performed with the patient supine. The examiner cradles the patient's chin and occiput, gently flexes the cervical spine, and applies a distracting force of up to 14 kg through the head and neck. If the symptoms in

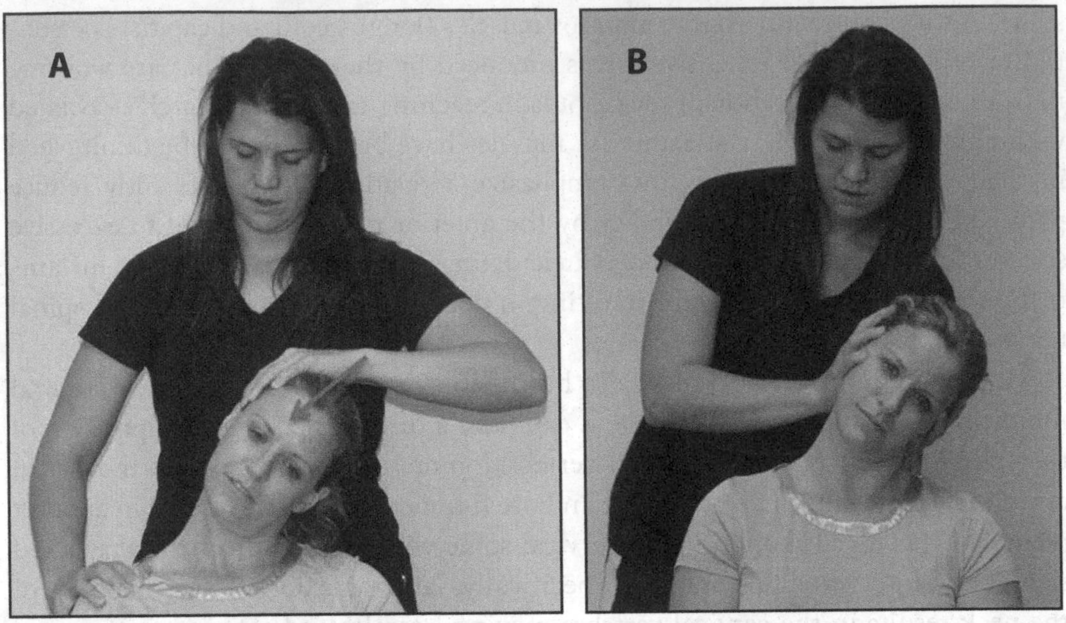

Figure 15-2. Spurling's test. (A) Compression force directed through the long axis of the neck as indicated by arrow. (B) Traction.

the upper extremity resolve, the result is positive. The upper limb tension test is performed with the patient supine. The examiner positions the patient close to the edge of the table so that his or her arm can be brought off the edge. The examiner slowly and sequentially moves the involved extremity into scapular depression, shoulder external rotation, abduction, forearm supination, wrist and finger extension, elbow extension, and, finally, cervical spine contralateral side-bending and rotation. If at any time during the movement the patient experiences pain that increases and radiates into the arm, the result is considered positive. If the examiner can move the arm equal to the uninvolved arm without reproducing symptoms, the result is negative. Range of motion can be measured using a goniometer or a cervical range of motion device. The shoulder abduction test has also been found to be moderately specific and sensitive, meaning it is moderately accurate as a positive test to rule in or a negative test to rule out cervical radiculopathy.[5] This test is simply performed by asking the patient to place the hand of his or her painful extremity on the top of his or her head. A positive result is relief of symptoms in the abducted position. If completion of these tests results in positive findings, follow-up would include performing further examination of light touch and pain sensation, reflexes, and muscle strength in the upper extremity at appropriate myotomal levels, which will assist in the identification of the specific spinal nerve root associated with the painful disorder.

References

1. Bono CM, Ghiselli G, Gilbert TJ, et al. An evidence-based clinical guideline for the diagnosis and treatment of cervical radiculopathy from degenerative disorders. *Spine J.* 2011;11(1):64-72.
2. O'Leary S, Falla D, Elliott JM, Jull G. Muscle dysfunction in cervical spine pain: implications for assessment and management. *J Orthop Sports Phys Ther.* 2009;39(5):324-333.
3. Neumann DA. *Kinesiology of the Musculoskeletal System: Foundations for Rehabilitation.* 2nd ed. St. Louis, MO: Mosby; 2009.
4. Wainner RS, Fritz JM, Irrgang JJ, Boninger ML, Delitto A, Allison S. Reliability and diagnostic accuracy of the clinical examination and patient self-report measures for cervical radiculopathy. *Spine.* 2003;28(1):52-62.
5. Ghasemi M, Golabchi K, Mousavi SA, et al. The value of provocative tests in diagnosis of cervical radiculopathy. *J Res Med Sci.* 2013;18(Suppl 1):S35-S38.

QUESTION **16**

What Mechanisms Contribute to Injury of the Peripheral Nerves at the Shoulder, and How Do These Injuries Present Clinically?

Lee N. Marinko, PT, ScD, OCS, FAAOMPT

Shoulder pain in the athlete can be the result of a nerve injury. Although nerve injuries are less common, early recognition of symptom behavior is necessary to prevent long-term disability. Injuries to nerves of the shoulder can occur from compression, stretching, or a combination. A transient stretch to the nerves in the upper extremity (a stinger) is a common occurrence in contact sports such as football, wrestling, and hockey. The most commonly described nerve compression disorders arise in the suprascapular, long thoracic, and axillary nerves. A clear understanding of each nerve's anatomical structure, mechanisms of compression or injury, and clinical presentation is fundamental. Outcomes of these injuries are variable and depend on the integrity of the neural axon and myelin sheath. The gold standard for diagnosis of any peripheral nerve entrapment is the use of electromyography (EMG) and nerve conduction velocity (NCV) testing, so any findings that present clinically as nerve injury should be followed up with subsequent testing for accurate diagnosis.

Huxel Bliven KC, ed. *Quick Questions in the Shoulder: Expert Advice in Sports Medicine* (pp 87-90).

Stingers, or transient episodes of radiating pain, weakness, and paresthesia, are thought to be an injury to either the cervical nerve roots or the brachial plexus and are addressed further in a subsequent chapter. Stingers are usually described as occurring with rapid lateral flexing of the neck with simultaneous depression of the scapula, as in a football tackle or wrestling pinning maneuver. Clinical findings usually occur within the spinal nerve distribution of C5 and C6, and sensory and motor loss may be present in the distal extremity.[1] The symptoms of this injury usually resolve spontaneously; however, the risk of reoccurrence is high. Continued monitoring of the athlete is necessary to prevent long-term neurovascular compromise.

The suprascapular nerve is the most commonly injured peripheral nerve in the athletic shoulder.[2] It arises from the upper trunk of the brachial plexus with contributions from the fifth and sixth spinal nerves. The nerve exits the plexus and travels laterally into the arm, passing posterior to the clavicle and anterior to the trapezius, just along the anterior border of the scapula. At the scapula, it passes through a small tunnel called the *suprascapular notch*. This tunnel can be variable but is most often described as being made up of the base of the coracoid process laterally and the transverse scapular ligament superiorly.[3] Once the nerve passes through the tunnel, it provides a motor branch to the supraspinatus muscle and sensory branches to the acromioclavicular and glenohumeral joints. It then continues along the spine of the scapula to the lateral edge, where it makes an almost 90-degree turn around the spinoglenoid tubercle to provide a motor branch into the infraspinatus muscle. The nerve can become entrapped at both the notch and the spinoglenoid tubercle. Extremes of scapular motion in repetitive overhead tasks, such as those in volleyball and tennis, can provoke traction and/or compression stresses to the nerve and result in injury. Compression to the nerve has also been described as arising from abnormal tissue adaptations or cysts secondary to labral or capsular injuries. Large tears in the posterior rotator cuff resulting in retracted muscle can also be the cause of a traction injury of this nerve.[4]

Individuals who sustain suprascapular injuries, whether in isolation or with concomitant shoulder injury, will describe symptoms such as a deep ache, a dull nonspecific pain in the superior aspect of the shoulder, or weakness with activity. Often, throwers or overhead athletes will describe a dead-arm feeling or loss of precision in their sport.[1,2] If the injury occurs proximally at the notch, motor function and atrophy may be seen in both the supraspinatus and infraspinatus muscles, and movement deficits can mimic those of a full-thickness rotator cuff tear. If the injury is distal to the spinoglenoid tubercle, the supraspinatus will be spared and motor deficits/atrophy will be present only in the infraspinatus (Figure 16-1).

The long thoracic nerve arises off the spinal nerve segments of C5, C6, and C7 and passes posterior to the brachial plexus down along the anterolateral thoracic cage.

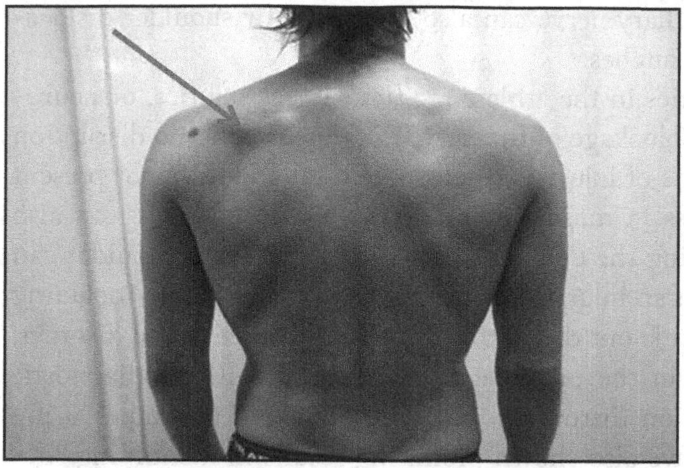

Figure 16-1. Suprascapular nerve injury. Note the atrophy in the right infraspinous fossa.

It is a pure motor nerve and innervates only the serratus anterior. It is, on average, 24 cm in length and can double this length with full elevation of the arm. Although not common, injury to this nerve can occur with traction to the neck or shoulder or with blunt trauma to the shoulder and has been reported in players of many sports, including tennis, archery, football, bowling, volleyball, weight-lifting, soccer, and hockey. Injury to this nerve is not usually associated with pain, but more commonly it presents as a disruption in scapula control with arm elevation. When the serratus is denervated, it can no longer maintain the scapula flush to the thorax, resulting in limited upward rotation of the scapula and excessive internal rotation (medial border elevation), commonly referred to as "winging." Patients may have impingement symptoms and weakness, specifically with overhead reaching.

The axillary nerve arises off the posterior trunk of the brachial plexus as one of the terminal branches with contributions from the fifth and sixth cervical nerve roots. The nerve travels inferolaterally on the anterior surface of the subscapularis muscle within the axilla and typically gives off motor branches to the anterior, middle, and posterior deltoid; the teres minor; and a sensory branch as the superior lateral cutaneous nerve.[5] It passes posteriorly through the quadrilateral space with the posterior circumflex artery. This space is bordered superiorly by the subscapularis and teres minor, inferiorly by the teres major, medially by the long head of the triceps, and laterally by the humerus. This nerve is susceptible to injury in the athlete at several sites, including where it arises from the posterior cord, the anterior inferior portion of the subscapularis muscle and glenohumeral joint capsule, the quadrilateral space, and within the fascicles of the deltoid muscles. The biomechanical demands that are placed on throwing or stick-handling athletes can produce both compressive or traction forces to this nerve over time. Symptoms of these injuries may be delayed in onset but may present as posterior shoulder pain and paresthesia over the lateral upper arm, with weakness in shoulder abduction and external rotation. The axillary nerve can also be injured by shoulder dislocation, trauma, or poor-fitting crutches.

Most peripheral nerve injuries in the athlete are first-degree injuries, or neuropraxias, that involve transient blockage of the nerve's conduction but no disruption to the neural sheath. This type of injury is often subclinical and does not present until there is a significant loss in muscle function. This type of injury can also be cumulative, so understanding the demands placed on an athlete's shoulder can help differentiate the causes of an injury. A comprehensive examination, including sensory and motor testing to rule out the cervical spine as a source of the disorder, should always be considered in the presence of such injuries. Electrodiagnostic studies will confirm conduction disruption and injury, but recent studies using musculoskeletal ultrasound have also shown promising results in identifying sites of entrapment.

References

1. Demertzis JL, Rubin DA. Upper extremity neuromuscular injuries in athletes. *Semin Musculoskelet Radiol.* 2012;16(4):316-330.
2. Brukner P, Khan K. *Brukner & Khan's Clinical Sports Medicine*. Sydney, Australia: McGraw Hill; 2011.
3. Moen TC, Babatunde OM, Hsu SH, Ahmad CS, Levine WN. Suprascapular neuropathy: what does the literature show? *J Shoulder Elbow Surg.* 2012;21(6):835-846.
4. Boykin RE, Friedman DJ, Higgins LD, Warner JJ. Suprascapular neuropathy. *J Bone Joint Surg Am.* 2010;92(13):2348-2364.
5. Loukas M, Grabska J, Tubbs RS, Apaydin N, Jordan R. Mapping the axillary nerve within the deltoid muscle. *Surg Radiol Anat.* 2009;31(1):43-47.

QUESTION 17

What Is the Role of Musculoskeletal Ultrasound in Diagnosing Shoulder Pathology?

Adam Lutz, PT, DPT and Chuck Thigpen, PhD, PT, ATC

The use of ultrasound imaging as a diagnostic tool for musculoskeletal pathologies has increased in prevalence in the past decade. As ultrasound is incorporated more frequently in the clinical setting, it is important to appraise the strengths and weaknesses of its use in conjunction with or in place of existing imaging modalities and clinical examination techniques. It is important to identify appropriate applications of diagnostic ultrasound and understand limitations that exist at this time in relation to shoulder pathology in the sports medicine setting.

Ultrasound imaging has demonstrated efficacy in evaluation of the bone morphology and many important characteristics of the muscles and tendons of the shoulder. Bony architecture of significance that can be evaluated via ultrasound imaging includes acromiohumeral distance (AHD) and humeral torsion. Measuring AHD is important because studies have demonstrated that small values of AHD are associated with large rotator cuff tears, superior migration of the humeral head, and poor surgical outcomes. Humeral torsion can be measured reliably using ultrasound imaging, and these measurements provide the clinician with

Huxel Bliven KC, ed. *Quick Questions in the Shoulder: Expert Advice in Sports Medicine* (pp 91-93).

important information in the development of a targeted intervention for patients with range of motion loss at the shoulder.

Ultrasound imaging can provide the clinician with vital information about musculotendinous characteristics such as disruptions (tears), muscle thickness or atrophy, fatty infiltration, and treatment effects.[1] Ultrasound has consistently demonstrated an ability to diagnose full-thickness rotator cuff tears that is equivalent to that of magnetic resonance imaging (MRI).[2] Muscle atrophy and fatty infiltration associated with chronic rotator cuff disease are assessed using the measurement of a cross-sectional area of the involved tissue. Higher levels of fatty infiltration affect intervention and are indicative of poor prognosis, and the quantity of fatty infiltration is closely correlated to the size of the rotator cuff tear.[3]

MRI and magnetic resonance arthrography (MRA) have long been relied on for diagnostic imaging of the shoulder but can be costly and time consuming. de Jesus et al[2] performed a meta-analysis that included 65 peer-reviewed articles and calculated the specificities and sensitivities of ultrasound imaging, MRI, and MRA compared with those of the gold standard of surgical findings. MRA was more sensitive and specific than MRI and ultrasound imaging, with a statistically significantly greater ability to detect full and partial tears, but there was no statistical difference between MRI and ultrasound. The authors concluded that "ultrasound may be the most cost-effective imaging method...for rotator cuff tears provided that the examiner has been properly trained in this operator-dependent technique."[2]

Ultrasound has been identified as an important imaging modality for the postoperative shoulder. As with the step-by-step tutorials that educate clinicians on thorough protocols for evaluations of the shoulder, publications exist that identify common surgical procedures of the shoulder and include discussions and examples of normal postoperative ultrasound images compared with those showing common postoperative complications. Miller et al[4] used serial ultrasound imaging to identify the rate and timing of re-tear after arthroscopic repair of large rotator cuff tears. In the rehabilitation setting, postoperative ultrasound can provide a skilled clinician with valuable information regarding tissue healing so that the patient can be appropriately managed based on tissue response.

Ultrasound is emerging as an important imaging modality in the sports medicine setting. It has been proven to be cost-effective, efficient, accurate, and well tolerated by patients for quantitative assessment of bone morphology and quantitative and qualitative evaluations of soft tissues of the shoulder. Experienced clinicians are able to quickly and efficaciously provide patients with vital information regarding their diagnosis, appropriate tissue-specific intervention, and prognosis. During postoperative assessments, clinicians are able to assess tissue recovery, appropriately progress the rehabilitation program based on healing, and identify stages of recovery in which the healing tissue is susceptible to failure. As this brief essay demonstrates, ultrasound imaging can be a valuable asset to the qualified sports medicine clinician. As with all diagnostic imaging and objective measurements, ultrasound imaging should be combined with the patient's overall clinical picture to develop the most appropriate intervention for the patient.

The primary limitation of the application of diagnostic ultrasound imaging for the shoulder is that it is highly dependent on the skill of the clinician who performs it. Thus, a clinician must be well trained and experienced in the use of ultrasound equipment and analyzing the imaging results. An experienced clinician is needed to provide the quality of images necessary to identify a tissue or structure as "normal" or "pathological" and, more importantly, whether the pathology is related to the patient's complaint. Several tutorials in the literature provide clinicians with step-by-step approaches to ensure comprehensive evaluation of the rotator cuff and shoulder in general and include detailed descriptions of normal tissues compared with abnormal tissues. Many of these publications provide the reader with information about common errors in administration of the ultrasound unit and analyses of the tissues being shown.[3,5]

References

1. Bailey LB, Shanley E, Fritz S, Seitz AL, Thigpen CA. Current concepts in rehabilitative ultrasound imaging of the shoulder: a clinical commentary. *J Orthop Sports Phys Ther.* In press.
2. de Jesus JO, Parker L, Frangos AJ, Nazarian LN. Accuracy of MRI, MR arthrography, and ultrasound in the diagnosis of rotator cuff tears: a meta-analysis. *AJR Am J Roentgenol.* 2009;192(6):1701-1707.
3. Beggs I. Shoulder ultrasound. *Semin Ultrasound CT MRI.* 2011;32(2):101-113.
4. Miller BS, Downie BK, Kohen RB, et al. When do rotator cuff repairs fail? Serial ultrasound examination after arthroscopic repair of large and massive rotator cuff tears. *Am J Sports Med.* 2011;39(10):2064-2070.
5. Jacobson JA. Shoulder US: anatomy, technique, and scanning pitfalls. *Radiology.* 2011; 260(1):6-16.

SECTION III

INJURY TREATMENT AND REHABILITATION

QUESTION 18

What Are the Best Patient-Rated Outcomes Measures for Use in Assessing Shoulder Pain and Dysfunction in Athletes?

Andréa Diniz Lopes, DSc and Eric L. Sauers, PhD, ATC, FNATA

Patient-rated outcomes (PRO) measures provide valuable information from the perspective of patients regarding their individual health status. Using PRO measures provides a means to assess the impact of sport-related injury pain and dysfunction on an individual's overall health. In addition, they can be used to evaluate the effectiveness of clinical interventions. PRO instruments are differentiated as either generic or specific measures. Generic outcomes instruments are multidimensional, cover a variety of domains of health-related quality of life (such as pain, impairments, functional limitations, and disability), and provide a broad view into a patient's health status.[1] Further, generic instruments allow for comparison of clinical outcomes across a spectrum of conditions (eg, compare between patient outcomes for lateral ankle sprains and shoulder instability). Specific outcomes instruments evaluate components of a patient's health status that may be affected by specific injuries, diseases, body regions, or injury sites and typically include questions that are highly relevant to that condition or region. For instance, if a

Huxel Bliven KC, ed. *Quick Questions in the Shoulder: Expert Advice in Sports Medicine* (pp 97-102).

certain impairment, such as night pain, is common for a specific condition, such as a rotator cuff tear, then a rotator cuff disease–specific instrument would most likely include items pertaining to night pain. Because of their specificity, specific outcomes measures are more responsive to changes in patients' perceptions of their health and better able to detect smaller differences resulting from particular interventions or exacerbations.

Recognizing the strengths and limitations of generic and specific outcomes is important when choosing the most appropriate PRO instruments for use in measuring an athlete's health status. In addition, it is also necessary to critically review available generic and specific instruments before implementing them in clinical practice. This is especially true with athletes, who have different physical demands and health-related values compared with those of the general population.[1] Athletes represent a distinct population because they mostly have a high physical functioning level and a high locus of internal control. Sport-related injuries that may not significantly alter a patient's ability to function in daily life may completely preclude him or her from participating in his or her chosen sport. Therefore, an athlete may achieve a normal score, demonstrating full function and health, on an outcome scale designed for the general population before he or she is able to achieve the full baseline physical function required for his or her sport. Therefore, ceiling effects of PRO measures designed for the general population are a significant concern with athletic populations.[2] Ceiling effects are a limitation of some instruments and occur when patients achieve a normal score on a PRO instrument despite having failed to achieve their full desired health status. Most generic and specific instruments were not developed for high-demand athletic patients; therefore, they fail to include items that are very important to this unique population. For example, many upper extremity region–specific scales ask patients about their ability to do things such as place a can on a high shelf, button a blouse, or perform self-care. These are important items for a 65-year-old patient with a massive rotator cuff tear. However, these items lack meaning and importance to a 22-year-old baseball pitcher who is unable to continue as a starter because of pain and functional loss caused by internal impingement.

There is a wide variety of PRO measures available with established measurement properties to assess shoulder function and disability, including disease- and region-specific scales.[3] The use of a disease-specific scale has great potential for evaluating specific domains affected by a target condition, but most disease-specific scales were not designed to measure conditions commonly observed in athletes. However, the Western Ontario Shoulder Instability Index (WOSI), designed to assess health-related quality of life in patients with shoulder instability, is a good example of a disease-specific outcome scale that could be used with athletes, because it is a common sport-related injury (Table 18-1). Although shoulder instability is

Table 18-1

Basic Characteristics of Recommended PRO Instruments Used for Athletes With Shoulder Pain and Dysfunction

Recommended Instrument	Type	Number of Subscales and Questions
SF-12	Generic	• 12 items • 2 subscales (physical health, mental health)
PSS	Region/joint specific; shoulder conditions including nonthrowing athletes	• 24 items • 3 subscales (pain, satisfaction, function)
DASH-SM	Region specific; upper extremity conditions including nonthrowing athletes	• 4 items • No subscales
WOSI	Disease specific; patients with instability	• 21 items • 4 subscales (physical symptoms, sports/recreation, lifestyle, emotions)
KJOC	Population and region specific; overhead throwing athletes	• 10 items • No subscales
FAST	Population and region specific; overhead throwing athletes	• 22 items • 5 subscales (throwing, advancement, pain, psychological, and activities of daily living) • Pitcher module (9 items)

a common condition in athletes, the WOSI was not designed specifically for athletes. Thus, while it contains questions that are pertinent for patients with instability, such as how much range of motion and looseness is present, a single sport-related question asks simply about the patient's ability to perform the specific skills required for sport or work. Therefore, despite producing a sports/recreation/work subscale score, this instrument does not capture a wide range of health-related information that would likely be considered important to high-demand athletic patients.

Although most of the specific outcomes instruments used for patients with shoulder conditions were designed for nonathlete patients, 2 have been extensively used in the literature and are recommended for nonthrowing athletes with shoulder pain and dysfunction: the Pennsylvania Shoulder Score (PSS) and the disabilities of the arm, shoulder, and hand (DASH) questionnaire (see Table 18-1).[3] The PSS is a shoulder-specific scale that provides information regarding shoulder pain level, function, and patient satisfaction. The DASH was designed for patients with various upper extremity conditions; it measures the patient's symptoms and ability to perform common daily and sports tasks via a separate DASH sports module (DASH-SM). The DASH-SM asks questions specifically related to the individual's sport participation, providing a measure of perceived sport function in nonthrowing athletes.[2,3] Few studies have assessed the use of PRO measures with athletic populations. Despite the fact that the DASH is generally recommended for athletes, it was shown to exhibit ceiling effects when used in college athletes with shoulder pain and injury. The presence of ceiling effects raises concerns regarding the instrument's validity for use with high-demand athletic shoulder patients. Until PRO instruments are developed for specific use with athletic populations, experts recommend the PSS and the DASH as the best available instruments for athletes with shoulder conditions.[3]

Overhead throwing athletes represent a special subset of athletic patients with unique demands and concerns because of the repetitive high forces inherent in their activity. Despite the general lack of PRO instruments designed for athletic populations, 2 region-specific scales were developed for assessing the health status of overhead throwing athletes with shoulder injuries. The Kerlan-Jobe Orthopaedic Clinic (KJOC) Shoulder and Elbow Questionnaire[4] is a specific PRO scale that was developed to assess functional ability and disability before and after shoulder and elbow injuries in overhead athletes (see Table 18-1). The KJOC contains items that are specific to throwers and is a valid and responsive instrument used to measure small changes in health status at the higher end of function in high-demand throwing athletes. The KJOC is a 10-item scale that is used predominantly to measure physical functioning and level of competition. The narrow focus of the KJOC requires that the clinician additionally administer a generic PRO instrument, such as the 12-Item Short Form Health Survey (SF-12; see Table 18-1), to more comprehensively assess global health status. The Functional Arm Scale for Throwers (FAST) is a second upper extremity region–specific PRO instrument developed for use in high-demand throwing populations (see Table 18-1).[5] The FAST is a 22-item scale designed to measure health-related quality of life after upper extremity injuries, without the need for administering a separate instrument. The FAST consists of an overall score and 5 subscales (throwing, advancement, pain, psychological, and activities of daily living), as well as a 9-item pitcher module, used only

Pitcher Module (All Pitchers MUST Complete this Section)

The following questions are to determine the impact of a baseball/softball pitchers arm injury on pitching-specific functional performance.

	Not at all	Slightly	Moderately	Severely	Unable to perform
1. How much has your arm injury limited the speed of your pitches?	1	2	3	4	5
2. How much has your arm injury limited your ability to throw 'bullpen' session?	1	2	3	4	5
3. How much has your arm injury limited your ability to 'hit' your spots?	1	2	3	4	5
4. How limited is your ability to pitch your turn in the rotation?	1	2	3	4	5
5. How much have your overall pitching statistics been hurt since your arm injury?	1	2	3	4	5
6. How much has your pitch count decreased since your arm injury?	1	2	3	4	5
7. How much has your arm injury limited your ability to throw different types of pitches?	1	2	3	4	5
8. Has your 'feel' for pitching decreased since your arm injury?	1	2	3	4	5
9. Do you need more time to recover between outings since your arm injury?	1	2	3	4	5

Figure 18-1. The FAST Pitcher Module with pitching specific questions designed to measure changes in health status at the highest levels of function. (Reprinted with permission from Eric L. Sauers, PhD, ATC, FNATA.)

with pitchers (Figure 18-1). However, caution should be used when interpreting the FAST because the responsiveness (or ability to detect changes over time) of the instrument is currently being assessed.

Choosing the most appropriate PRO instrument for athletes with shoulder pain and dysfunction is a significant clinical challenge given the high functional level of this particular population of patients. For nonthrowing athletes with shoulder pain and dysfunction, we recommend the PSS and DASH-SM scales. These instruments provide clinicians and patients with valuable information regarding the impact of the patient's shoulder injury or condition on his or her health status and can be used to measure change in health over time. Caution is recommended because of the potential for ceiling effects, especially during the latter stages of rehabilitation as patients are transitioning back into sports participation but may still be suffering from pain and functional limitations that are too subtle for these instruments to detect. For overhead throwing athletes, we recommend using either the KJOC or the FAST. At this time, the KJOC is recommended over the FAST for measuring changes in health status over time, because the responsiveness of this instrument has been demonstrated. However, the addition of a generic health status measure is recommended when using the KJOC.

References

1. Parsons JT, Snyder AR. Health-related quality of life as a primary clinical outcome in sport rehabilitation. *J Sport Rehabil.* 2011;20(1):17-36.
2. Hsu JE, Nacke E, Park MJ, Sennett BJ, Huffman GR. The Disabilities of the Arm, Shoulder, and Hand questionnaire in intercollegiate athletes: validity limited by ceiling effect. *J Shoulder Elbow Surg.* 2010;19(3):349-354.
3. Thigpen C, Shanley E. Clinical assessment of upper extremity injury outcomes. *J Sport Rehabil.* 2011;20(1):61-73.
4. Alberta FG, ElAttrache NS, Bissell S, et al. The development and validation of a functional assessment tool for the upper extremity in the overhead athlete. *Am J Sports Med.* 2010;38(5):903-911.
5. Sauers EL, Dykstra DL, Bay RC, Bliven KH, Snyder AR. Upper extremity injury history, current pain rating, and health-related quality of life in female softball pitchers. *J Sport Rehabil.* 2011;20(1):100-114.

QUESTION 19

What Strategies Can Be Implemented to Integrate Patient-Rated Outcomes Measures Into the Routine Care of Patients With Shoulder Injury?

Alison R. Snyder Valier, PhD, AT, FNATA

Routine collection of patient outcomes is a consistent health care initiative. While there has been great emphasis on evaluating patient outcomes through the use of patient-rated outcomes (PRO) instruments, there has been little guidance on how best to implement them into patient care. Giving someone a survey to complete seems like an easy task, but there are some things to consider before implementation so that a successful strategy is created and meaningful and useful information is obtained from patients.

Before implementing a PRO instrument, it is important to consider your purpose and what type of information you wish to gather from the patient.[1] In general, PRO instruments can be classified as either generic or specific.[2-4] Generic measures provide a more global, general evaluation of health status than specific measures, which naturally makes them lack specificity for, and potentially relevance to, any one injury or body region, such as the shoulder.[2-4] In contrast, specific instruments are highly relevant to specific injuries or body regions because their questions are

Huxel Bliven KC, ed. *Quick Questions in the Shoulder: Expert Advice in Sports Medicine* (pp 103-107).

tailored to people with those conditions.[2-4] The narrow, targeted focus of specific instruments makes them more likely to respond to treatments and interventions than generic instruments. Ideally, both generic and specific instruments should be completed by patients because of the different types of information captured by them. When creating an outcomes collection strategy, it is important to determine the type of information you wish to obtain because content should be one criterion that drives instrument selection.

Another consideration is the length of the instrument. The simplest PRO instruments contain only one question. Single-item instruments tend to address global concepts such as pain, function, and satisfaction and are easy to complete, score, and interpret. Multi-item instruments, in contrast, provide a more robust evaluation of an injury or a health construct and evaluate one, or commonly several, dimensions of health that provide a greater depth of information about the impact of an injury on the specific health dimension. One of the most often-reported barriers to the use of PRO instruments is time to administer, complete, and score,[5] which may be more of an issue when considering multi- vs single-item measures. Therefore, clinicians should weigh the trade-offs between depth of information obtained and time to administer when choosing between shorter and longer PRO instruments.

Once you have determined the type of information desired (generic, specific, or both) and the length of instrument that can be accommodated in your facility, it is necessary to identify a strategy for implementation. Unfortunately, there is no one-size-fits-all approach for the collection of PRO measures. There are, however, some suggestions for different ways you can approach the assessment of patient outcomes, which we term *simple*, *standard*, and *patient-centered strategies*.

A simple strategy is just that—simple. The goal of a simple strategy is to initiate the collection of patient outcomes routinely, and the simplest way to meet this goal is to implement 1 or 2 single-item outcomes instruments into your clinical practice. For example, on a routine basis, you can administer the single assessment numeric evaluation (SANE), which allows patients to grade their injury on a scale from 1 to 100 at each patient visit (Figure 19-1). Additionally, after the first visit, you might consider evaluating the change that patients perceive they have experienced by asking them to complete the global rating of change (GROC) (Figure 19-2). Although these 2 instruments provide only a snapshot of overall health status, they do allow you to begin to systematically and objectively capture patient-perceived health status and change in health status over time. The value in serial administration of PRO, even using single-item instruments, is that you not only objectively capture patient voice but you can also begin to measure the effectiveness of the treatments and interventions you deliver and use the information to support patient care decisions.

If I had to give my shoulder a grade from 1 to 100, with 100 being the best, I would give my shoulder a ______.

Figure 19-1. Single-Item Numeric Evaluation (SANE).

Please rate the overall condition of your shoulder from the time that you began treatment until now (check only one):		
___A great deal worse (-3)	___No Change (0)	___A great deal better (+3)
___Somewhat worse (-2)		___Somewhat better (2)
___Slightly worse (-1)		___Slightly better (1)

Figure 19-2. Global Rating of Change (GROC).

The second suggested approach is the standardized strategy. The standardized strategy is similar to the simple strategy for collecting PRO measures, but instead of restricting yourself to single-item instruments, you standardize the use of single- and multi-item instruments across your patients. Ideally, you should select both a generic and a specific instrument so that you can evaluate overall health status and health status more specifically related to the injury. Standardizing instruments takes the guesswork out of what to use with your patients and should save time. For example, all patients, regardless of shoulder injury, could receive the disablement in the physically active scale (DPAS) as your generic measure of outcome. The selection of specific instruments would be standardized to injury, body region, or athlete type. For example, if you see a high volume of throwing athletes with shoulder conditions, you could administer a specific instrument that was developed for that population, such as the Functional Arm Scale for Throwers (FAST) or the Kerlan-Jobe Orthopaedic Clinic (KJOC) scale. Nonthrowing athletes, then, would receive a different shoulder-specific instrument, such as the Pennsylvania Shoulder Score (PSS). Your standardized approach, with this scenario, would result in all patients with a shoulder condition receiving the same generic instrument (the DPAS), throwers receiving the FAST or KJOC, and nonthrowers receiving the PSS. The key with the standardized approach is that you select the instruments based on the specific injury, body region, or athlete type and not on the individual patient case. The standardized approach should save time because the instruments are preselected. In addition, by administering the same instrument to similar types of patients, all of the outcomes from this group of patients could be evaluated and compared, which would provide valuable information about the effectiveness of treatments and interventions.

A final strategy is to select PRO instruments based on the specific needs of the patient, and because the focus is on the patient, we call this the patient-centered approach. Unlike the simple and standardized strategies, the patient-centered approach necessitates attention to the specific patient case and selection of instruments to meet the needs of that patient. Like with the standardized approach, the recommendation is to include both generic and specific instruments, but the choice of those instruments may vary from patient to patient. For a patient who has trouble with pain and function, you may select the PSS because it includes 3 questions on pain and a number of questions related to function, whereas you might opt to select the disabilities of the arm, shoulder, and hand (DASH) questionnaire when disability is the primary concern. Using a patient-centered approach provides the best opportunity to deliver care that targets the specific needs of the patient and should inform and support clinical decisions. However, when choice of instrument is not standardized, it is not as easy to compare outcomes between or across different patients or between clinicians because the measurement tools are not the same. Over time, it is likely that you will use similar instruments enough across patients to make comparisons, but it likely would take longer to do so with the patient-centered approach than with a standardized approach.

Once you select the strategy that best fits your situation, identifying a timeline for serial administration is important. Like with the selection of instruments, there is no one-size-fits-all timeline approach, and outcomes can be delivered at any point in care. It may be helpful, though, to consider some consistent time points so that the time of administration becomes routine, making it easy to remember to implement. At a minimum, the first and last (eg, discharge and return-to-play) patient care visits are captured because you can evaluate the change you have made in the patient's health status from the start to the end of care. Including additional administrations between the start and end is suggested because these time points allow the information you obtained from the PRO measure to affect clinical decisions. Midpoint outcomes measures reflecting perceived patient improvement may suggest continuation of the current patient care plan, whereas midpoint assessments indicating the perception of no change or poorer health status may suggest altering the care plan. It is important to note that many PRO instruments have recall periods of 1 or more weeks, and it is suggested that those times be avoided for reassessment of outcomes. Tables 19-1 and 19-2 provide examples of administration strategies. Note that any combination of instruments can be administered during these time points. Another component essential to the successful implementation and use of PRO instruments is an understanding of common measures of change, such as clinically important change, which is the smallest amount of change a patient perceives as beneficial. These values are the basis for determining change in patient health status over time.

Although using PRO instruments to support health care decision making is not new, their use is not widespread. The purpose of the suggestions provided here is

Table 19-1

Example Time Points for Administration of PRO Instruments at First and Final Visits

Instrument	First Visit	Last Visit
SANE	X	X
GROC		X

Table 19-2

Example Time Points for Serial Administration of PRO Instruments Over Multiple Visits

Instrument	First Visit	Week 2	Week 4	Last Visit
DPAS	X			X
FAST	X	X	X	X
SANE	X	X	X	X
GROC				X

to present strategies for overcoming barriers to their implementation, such as time, and to develop small steps to feasible and successful use of PRO instruments in clinical settings.

References

1. Snyder AR, Valovich McLeod TC. Selecting patient-based outcome measures. *Athl Ther Today.* 2007;12(6):12-15.
2. Fitzpatrick R, Davey C, Buxton MJ, Jones DR. Evaluating patient-based outcome measures for use in clinical trials. *Health Technol Assess.* 1998;2(14):i-iv, 1-74.
3. Suk M, Hanson BP, Norvell DC, Helfet DL. *Musculoskeletal Outcomes Measures and Instruments.* Vol 1. Davos, Switzerland: AO Publishing; 2009.
4. Valovich McLeod TC, Snyder AR, Parsons JT, Curtis Bay R, Michener LA, Sauers EL. Using disablement models and clinical outcomes assessment to enable evidence-based athletic training practice, part II: clinical outcomes assessment. *J Athl Train.* 2008;43(4):437-445.
5. Snyder Valier AR, Jennings AL, Parsons JT, Vela LI. Benefits of and barriers to using patient-rated outcome measures in athletic training. *J Athl Train.* 2014;49(5):674-683.

QUESTION 20

What Factors Should Be Considered in the Early Management of a First-Time Traumatic Anterior Shoulder Dislocation?

Kellie C. Huxel Bliven, PhD, ATC

Anterior glenohumeral (GH) joint dislocations are classified as traumatic and atraumatic, and each type has its own course of care. Traumatic GH joint dislocations account for more than 90% of shoulder dislocations and are often associated with fractures, rotator cuff injury, and neurological complications.[1] Populations that account for the highest proportion of traumatic GH joint dislocations are individuals aged 20 to 30 years (~25%), males (2.5 times more likely than females), and contact sport athletes.[2] After a first-time traumatic anterior GH joint dislocation, a primary goal should be to identify the most effective treatment to reduce the likelihood of recurrence. This chapter will examine and recommend strategies for clinicians to consider in the management of a first-time traumatic anterior GH joint dislocation.

Traditionally, GH joint dislocations have been treated with a course of nonsurgical care, including immobilization, followed by a rehabilitation program. Nonsurgical care is considered a failure if the patient experiences an instability episode within 2 years of the initial dislocation and subsequently undergoes surgical

Huxel Bliven KC, ed. *Quick Questions in the Shoulder: Expert Advice in Sports Medicine* (pp 109-111).

stabilization with relative success. High recurrence rates with the nonsurgical management approach have prompted discussion and research on effective management techniques for individuals with a first-time traumatic anterior GH joint dislocation.

In general, the management of a traumatic anterior GH dislocation has included immobilization in a position of adduction and internal rotation for a period of 2 to 6 weeks. This strategy has been challenged by studies that demonstrated significantly lower recurrence rates when the immobilization position was abduction and external rotation.[1-3] The basis for this immobilization position is twofold: (1) external rotation up to 45 degrees centers the humeral head within the glenoid labrum and, in doing so, promotes tissue approximation for optimal healing; and (2) the subscapularis is lengthened and taut in external rotation, which reduces hematoma formation and further improves tissue approximation.[4] Although the results of biomechanical and cadaveric studies support these theories, there is conflicting evidence-based research regarding the immobilization position that yields the lowest recurrence rates. Until recently, some of the discrepancy was attributed to poor-quality studies with a bias that affected the generalizability of the results. Unfortunately, current studies involving randomized, controlled trials and systematic reviews of better-quality studies have still not provided clarity regarding the most effective immobilization position.[1,3,4] Future research may provide insight about management practices if populations are stratified by age, sex, activity level, and tissue damage (eg, Bankart lesion, bone lesion).[3,4] To date, evidence does not support the use of one position as superior for reducing recurrence rates.

Other factors to consider regarding immobilization are the optimal amount of external rotation and duration for achieving the best outcomes. The exact amount of external rotation has not been defined. Results of cadaver studies suggest that 45 degrees of external rotation is optimal; however, this position is uncomfortable for patients, and compliance rates have been poor.[1,3] Therefore, it is recommended that external rotation between 10 and 15 degrees be used to increase compliance rates and improve healing. Another factor that must be considered is the length of time the patient is immobilized. There is a balance between immobilization duration to achieve tissue healing and excessive immobilization that can negatively affect mobility and function. Research suggests that a 3-week immobilization period is optimal after a first-time traumatic anterior GH joint dislocation.[1] Shorter than 3 weeks did not allow adequate time for tissue approximation and healing; longer than 3 weeks resulted in a significant decrease in patient compliance and no added benefits with regard to reduced recurrence rates.

The high proportion of traumatic anterior GH dislocations and recurrences in male contact sport participants younger than 30 years has led to focused study of this at-risk population. Although nonsurgical treatments continue to be the standard management for a first-time traumatic anterior GH joint dislocation, there is evidence to suggest that young male athletes have better functional outcomes if they initially undergo surgical stabilization rather than nonsurgical care.[3] Furthermore, recurrence rates reported in a recent systematic review were significantly lower in the surgical stabilization group (9.6% to 27%) than in the nonsurgical treatment group (37.5%).[3] Interestingly, a comparison of the cost-effectiveness of a primary arthroscopic stabilization procedure, including postsurgical rehabilitation, with the expenses for a course of nonsurgical care determined that the costs were greater for nonsurgical management because it was often unsuccessful and surgical stabilization became necessary.[5] The surgical route immediately after a first-time anterior GH joint dislocation not only produced better functional outcomes in young adults, but cost less overall.[5] As such, clinicians should not discount surgical stabilization as a viable option following a first-time dislocation, especially if the patient is a young adult and an athlete.

Clinicians should be aware of the effect of immobilization position and duration after first-time anterior GH dislocation on injury recurrence. Researchers are currently unable to strongly recommend immobilization in abduction and external rotation over adduction and internal rotation; however, as study designs are refined to address a specific age or population, treatment options may expand. In addition, surgical intervention should be considered an option in managing a first-time anterior GH joint dislocation.

References

1. Heidari K, Asadollahi S, Vafaee R, et al. Immobilization in external rotation combined with abduction reduces the risk of recurrence after primary anterior shoulder dislocation. *J Shoulder Elbow Surg*. 2014;23(6):759-766.
2. Murray IR, Ahmed I, White NJ, Robinson CM. Traumatic anterior shoulder instability in the athlete. *Scand J Med Sci Sports*. 2013;23(4):387-405.
3. Longo UG, Loppini M, Rizzello G, Ciuffreda M, Maffulli N, Denaro V. Management of primary acute anterior shoulder dislocation: systematic review and quantitative synthesis of the literature. *Arthroscopy*. 2014;30(4):506-522.
4. Vavken P, Sadoghi P, Quidde J, et al. Immobilization in internal or external rotation does not change recurrence rates after traumatic anterior shoulder dislocation. *J Shoulder Elbow Surg*. 2014;23(1):13-19.
5. Crall TS, Bishop JA, Guttman D, Kocher M, Bozic K, Lubowitz JH. Cost-effectiveness analysis of primary arthroscopic stabilization versus nonoperative treatment for first-time anterior glenohumeral dislocations. *Arthroscopy*. 2012;28(12):1755-1765.

QUESTION 21

Which Types of Acromioclavicular Joint Separations Respond Best to Nonoperative Management, and What Rehabilitation Guidelines Ensure a Safe Return to Play?

Michael A. Shaffer, PT, ATC, OCS

There are several classification systems used to describe acromioclavicular (AC) joint injury. Clinicians should be aware of the classifications, involved structures, and management recommendations for each level of severity to make the most appropriate treatment and return-to-play decisions. The 6 types of AC sprains described by Rockwood will serve as the classification scheme used in this chapter (Table 21-1).[1] Type I and II injuries involve the AC ligaments and do not produce significant superior displacement of the clavicle. Type III injuries include damage to the AC ligaments and the coracoclavicular (CC) ligaments. Rupture of the CC ligaments results in the step-off deformity of the clavicle that is pathognomonic for AC joint separation. Type IV to VI injuries are those with even more profound displacement of the distal clavicle than is present with Type III injuries. The extent of clavicular displacement is such that Type IV to VI injuries require surgical stabilization. Typically, Type I to III injuries respond well to conservative management.[2]

Huxel Bliven KC, ed. *Quick Questions in the Shoulder: Expert Advice in Sports Medicine* (pp 113-117).

Table 21-1

Rockwood Classification System for Acromioclavicular Joint Sprains[a]

Type	AC Joint Status	CC Ligament Status	CC Interspace Distance	Deltotrapezial Fascia
I	Sprain	Intact	Normal	Intact
II	Complete injury	Sprain	Slightly more than normal	Intact
III	Complete injury	Complete injury	Increased <100%	Intact
IV	Complete injury	Complete injury	Variable injury	Torn
V	Complete injury	Complete injury	100% to 300% increase	Torn
VI	Complete injury	Intact/sprain	Less than normal	Variable injury

[a]Common to all injuries is partial or complete disruption of the AC joint. Complete disruption of the AC joint distinguishes Type I from Type II. Complete disruption of the CC ligaments (allowing for clear radiographic AC separation) distinguishes Type II from III. Greater degrees (> 100% increased separation) of distal clavicle elevation (or acromial depression) with disruption of the deltotrapezial fascia and subsequent closed irreducibility of the AC joint distinguishes Type III from Type V. Posterior displacement of the distal clavicle through the deltotrapezial fascia identifies a Type IV injury. Type VI injuries are rare hyperabduction injuries in which the distal clavicle comes to lie under the coracoid, with inherent neurovascular injury risk.

Reprinted with permission from Gaunt BW, McCluskey GM, eds. *A Systematic Approach to Shoulder Rehabilitation.* Columbus, GA: Human Performance and Rehabilitation Centers; 2012.

Figure 21-1. Photograph demonstrating an American football player about to land directly on his acromion (ie, the "point" of the shoulder), a common mechanism of injury causing AC separations. (Reprinted with permission from Brian Roy.)

Most AC sprains occur when an athlete directly lands on the "point" of the shoulder (the acromion; Figure 21-1). An athlete is particularly vulnerable to AC joint injury when he or she is unable to brace for the fall, such as during biking with hands left on the handlebars or in American football when a runner is tackled with the arms pinned to the sides.[2] AC joint injury can also occur with a fall onto the outstretched hand or contact with an opponent during blocking, tackling, or checking. Rugby, wrestling, and hockey are collegiate sports for which a high incidence of AC sprains is reported. Male cadets at West Point had a 2.2-times-higher incidence of injury than female cadets.[3] In a review of the National Collegiate Athletic Association injury database for American football, AC injuries accounted for 4.5% of all injuries, and contact with an opponent produced 72% of AC joint injuries, with 48% occurring when tackling or being tackled.[4]

Less severe AC joint sprains are more frequent than higher-energy injuries that result in more severe pathology. Type I and II AC injuries accounted for 96% of all AC joint injuries in collegiate athletes.[4] Because vertical stability of the AC joint is maintained by the CC ligaments, there is no gross displacement with Type I and II AC joint sprains. Therefore, the focus of rehabilitation for these sprains should be placed on restoring full and pain-free shoulder girdle range of motion followed by restoring strength. Full shoulder flexion requires elevation and rotation of the clavicle. Consequently, end-range shoulder flexion is often painful and initially limited after injury. However, forward flexion generally returns more quickly than cross-body adduction (CBA) range of motion, which places superior stresses on the clavicle as it is compressed against the acromion. Active assisted and passive range of motion exercises (eg, supine elevation with an exercise wand) are helpful in restoring AC joint motion, whereas CBA motions are best avoided during rehabilitation. Rather than target CBA with therapeutic exercises, one strategy is

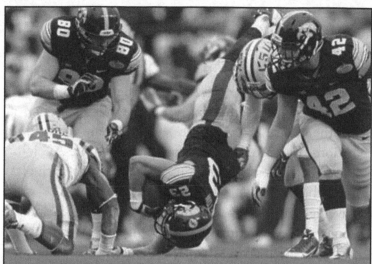

to monitor the athlete to ensure that CBA motion is returning and to use pain or limitation as an indicator to determine the need for continued rehabilitation or approval for return to activity/play.

Rotator cuff and periscapular strengthening are believed to be beneficial in helping minimize stresses on the healing ligaments around the AC joint. These exercises are begun with the arm down by the side, limiting range of motion as necessary because of pain. As the athlete recovers, these exercises are moved into more elevated/end-range positions. Because of the stresses placed on the AC joint, chest press, bench press, and overhead press (eg, military press) are among the last exercises to be added during rehabilitation.[5]

In collegiate football, the average time lost is 11.6 days for Type I and II sprains and 31.9 days for Type III injuries.[4] Approximately 8% to 42% of athletes with Type I or II injuries will have long-term symptoms. If radiographs indicate subsequent degeneration of the AC joint, corticosteroid injections or distal clavicle excision may be an option.[5]

Type III AC injuries include the superior elevation of the clavicle that is pathognomonic for AC joint sprains. Athletes with an AC joint sprain, particularly those with superior displacement of the clavicle, may benefit from the short-term use of a standard sling to unload the arm. Despite the obvious loss of AC joint integrity with superior displacement of the clavicle, the vast majority of athletes with Type III AC injuries still do quite well with conservative management.[2] Athletes with Type III injuries are typically able to regain full strength and range of motion despite the remaining deformity. If symptoms persist during tackling or blocking, an athlete with Type III injuries might require modification of his or her shoulder pads or a custom thermoplastic orthosis to help protect the AC joint. A small percentage (22%) of patients with Type III injuries remain symptomatic and will eventually undergo surgical reconstruction.[4] Athletes with a Type III AC sprain typically undergo rehabilitation for 3 to 6 months before the decision is made about whether to pursue surgical stabilization.

Type IV and V AC injuries are characterized by the clavicle displacing through the deltotrapezial fascia. Type VI injuries occur when the clavicle is displaced inferiorly and lodged behind the conjoined tendon of the biceps and/or coracobrachialis. Because of the inherent instability of the AC joint and potential injury to surrounding soft tissues that a displaced, mobile distal clavicle may cause, athletes with a Type IV, V, or VI AC joint injury typically undergo surgical stabilization.[5] Some surgeons perform stabilization with anatomic reconstruction of the AC and CC ligaments with a semitendinosus autograft. Sling immobilization is typically maintained for at least 6 weeks. Because Type IV to VI AC joint injuries are rare, rehabilitation of these conditions is even more unlikely. As such, the postoperative rehabilitation program is not described here.

Conclusion

AC joint injuries occur most commonly in collision sports. Type I and II injuries, which primarily damage the AC ligaments, are most common. Type III injuries involve the AC and CC ligaments and are indicated by superior displacement of the clavicle. Despite the obvious loss of AC joint integrity, most athletes with a Type III injury, similar to those with a Type I or II injury, typically do very well with a period of rehabilitation. By contrast, athletes with more severe injuries (Type IV to VI), indicated by significant loss of alignment of the distal clavicle, typically require surgical stabilization even for activities of daily living.

Acknowledgment

The author thanks Jimmy Boeckenstedt, ATS-3, University of Iowa, for his assistance.

References

1. Gaunt BW, McCluskey GM, eds. *A Systematic Approach to Shoulder Rehabilitation*. Columbus, GA: Human Performance and Rehabilitation Centers; 2012.
2. Johansen JA, Grutter PW, McFarland EG, Petersen SA. Acromioclavicular joint injuries: indications for treatment and treatment options. *J Shoulder Elbow Surg*. 2011;20(2 Suppl):S70-S82.
3. Pallis M, Cameron KL, Svoboda SJ, Owens BD. Epidemiology of acromioclavicular joint injury in young athletes. *Am J Sports Med*. 2012;40(9):2072-2077.
4. Dragoo JL, Braun HJ, Bartlinski SE, Harris AH. Acromioclavicular joint injuries in National Collegiate Athletic Association football: data from the 2004-2005 through 2008-2009 National Collegiate Athletic Association Injury Surveillance System. *Am J Sports Med*. 2012;40(9):2066-2071.
5. Rios CG, Mazzocca AD. Acromioclavicular joint problems in athletes and new methods of management. *Clin Sports Med*. 2008;27(4):763-788.

QUESTION 22

After a Brachial Plexopathy, What Are the Most Important Considerations for Determining When an Athlete Can Safely Return to Collision and Contact Sports?

Michael A. Shaffer, PT, ATC, OCS

Unilateral transient brachial plexopathy (a stinger or burner) occurs when the brachial plexus is traumatically stretched, compressed, or contused, resulting in symptoms of tingling or warmth into the upper part of the arm (Figure 22-1).[1] This injury occurs most commonly when the athlete is trying to tackle or block an opponent and has a forceful separation of the head and shoulder (Figure 22-2). This position places traction stress on the C5-C6 nerve roots and the upper trunk of the brachial plexus contralateral to the side of the head displacement. In addition, excessive lateral flexion produces compression forces on the nerve roots ipsilateral to the direction of the head. Some authors have postulated that traction injuries are more common in young athletes, whereas compressive lesions are more common in collegiate and professional athletes.[7]

Stingers are most common in collision sports, including American football, rugby, and Australian rules football, which require tackling or blocking an opponent. It has been reported that 50% to 65% of collegiate football players will

Huxel Bliven KC, ed. *Quick Questions in the Shoulder: Expert Advice in Sports Medicine* (pp 119-122).

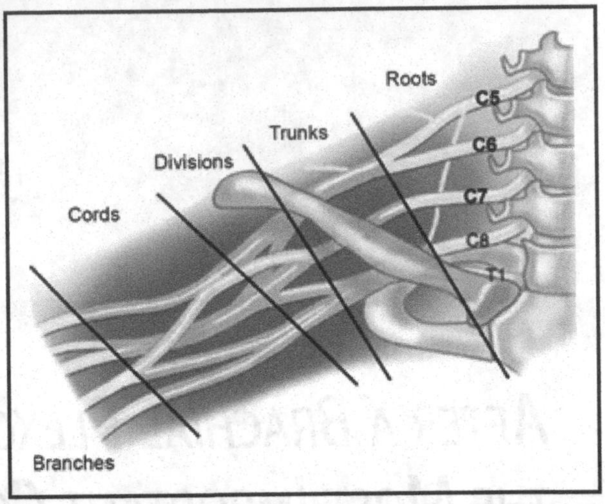

Figure 22-1. Brachial plexus. (Reprinted with permission from Gaunt BW, McCluskey GM III, eds. *A Systematic Approach to Shoulder Rehabilitation.* Columbus, GA: Human Performance and Rehabilitation Centers, Inc; 2012.)

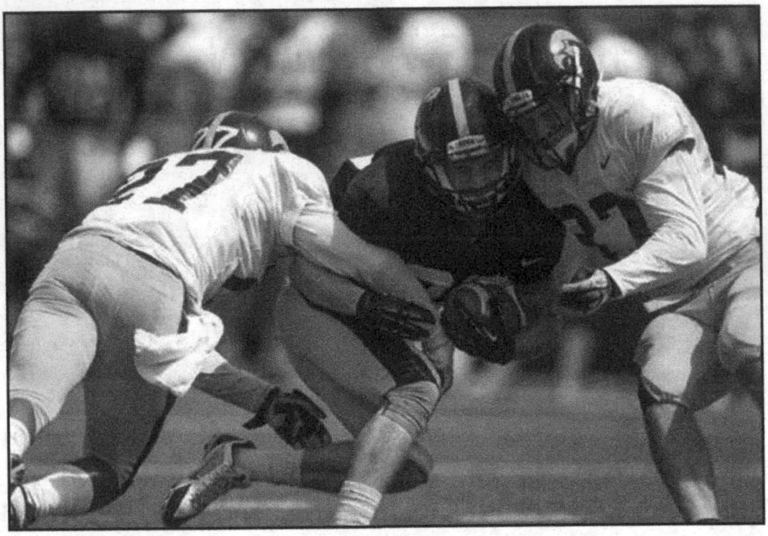

Figure 22-2. Photograph demonstrating the forceful lateral flexion of the neck that can occur when making a tackle or being tackled during American football practice. (Reprinted with permission from Brian Roy.)

suffer a stinger during their career.[2] In fact, athletes with more years of playing experience, particularly those who play the position of linebacker or on the offensive or defensive lines, have a higher incidence of injury.[3]

The neurologic symptoms associated with a stinger are typically transient and resolve within seconds or minutes. Rapid resolution allows the athlete to return to the same practice or competition, but the on-site medical personnel must determine the timing of return to play. Stingers can become a recurrent problem. In general, the more recurrent the injury, the longer the time for symptoms to resolve and strength to return.[1]

Athletes who sustain a stinger often display typical patterns or movements in response to the stinging or burning sensations. Most athletes remove themselves from competition and hold their arm to their side, motionless—the characteristic "dead arm"—or, conversely, shake their arm in an effort to alleviate the sensations.

As the head is laterally flexed forcefully, the nerves of the brachial plexus are stretched or compressed, putting stress on the myelin sheath that covers the outside of the nerve, which results in a low-level injury to the sheath while sparing the underlying nerve tissue. In terms of Seddon's classification of nerve injury, a stinger would be labeled a neuropraxia, which explains the temporary nature and, in the vast majority of cases, the full recovery of nerve function within seconds or minutes.[1]

Because the C5-C6 nerve roots are usually affected, muscles supplied within these myotomes (eg, biceps, deltoid, and external rotators of the shoulder) may demonstrate profound weakness. Muscle testing should be repeated every 3 to 5 minutes to determine if the athlete has regained full strength, which is necessary for return to competition. Full return of strength confirms only mild injury to the neurologic tissues and allows the athlete to safely and effectively return to his or her sport. In addition, medical personnel should ensure that the athlete has regained full cervical range of motion and has a negative Spurling test result. In the majority of cases, symptoms resolve within minutes. However, weakness may linger occasionally, particularly in severe or repeated injuries. In these cases, a rehabilitation program of strengthening is often performed for affected muscle groups. If weakness persists for 2 weeks or more, advanced imaging and electrodiagnostic testing may be necessary.[2]

Once an athlete sustains a stinger, particularly a compressive lesion, there is an increased chance of sustaining another stinger.[3] From a physical standpoint, strengthening of the cervical muscles is the primary form of prevention because stronger neck muscles are better able to resist external loads to the head and neck. Perhaps the best prevention is blocking or tackling with proper technique to avoid separation of the head and shoulder.[1] In addition, in American football, neck rolls or pads can be added to the shoulder pads, which limit excessive cervical side-bending and extension. In general, the more repetitive the injury, the greater time will be required for symptoms to resolve and strength to return.

A risk factor for recurrent stingers that cannot be addressed through rehabilitation is the relative size of the spinal cord to the diameter of the vertebral foramen (the mean subaxial cervical space available for the cord [MSCSAC]).[4] Previously, Torg identified a ratio of the diameter of the vertebral foramen relative to the width of the vertebral body that was predictive for recurrent stingers. However, the MSCSAC is thought to be a more accurate predictor because the ratio is averaged over the C3-C6 spinal levels. A ratio of less than 4.3 mm translates to the athlete being 13 times more likely to experience chronic stingers.[4] The obvious disadvantage to using the MSCSAC is that it requires an MRI examination to measure the diameter of the spinal cord, whereas the Torg ratio can be calculated from standard radiographs.

Conclusion

Stingers occur most commonly in collision sports, particularly those that involve blocking or tackling. These actions can produce a compression or traction injury on the upper portions of the brachial plexus. The forces injure the myelin sheath, which typically results in transient sensations of stinging and burning into the C5-C6 dermatomes, with concomitant weakness of the biceps, deltoid, and shoulder external rotators. Return to play is permitted when strength, as assessed by manual muscle testing, is symmetric, the burning/stinging symptoms have resolved, and full cervical range of motion is demonstrated.[2] Athletes with repeated stingers should strengthen their neck muscles, re-evaluate their tackling technique, and have additional padding attached to their shoulder pads to limit excessive cervical extension and lateral flexion. If stingers become recurrent, imaging studies to assess the patency of the athlete's intervertebral foramen and available space for the spinal cord may be warranted.

Acknowledgment

The author thanks Jimmy Boeckenstedt, ATS-3, University of Iowa, for his assistance.

References

1. Weinberg J, Rokito S, Silber JS. Etiology, treatment, and prevention of athletic "stingers." *Clin Sports Med.* 2003;22(3):493-500.
2. Standaert CJ, Herring SA. Expert opinion and controversies in musculoskeletal and sports medicine: stingers. *Arch Phys Med Rehabil.* 2009;90(3):402-406.
3. Charbonneau RM, McVeigh SA, Thompson K. Brachial neuropraxia in Canadian Atlantic University sport football players: what is the incidence of "stingers"? *Clin J Sports Med.* 2012;22(6):472-477.
4. Presciutti SM, DeLuca P, Marchetto P, Wilsey JT, Shaffrey C, Vaccaro AR. Mean subaxial space available for the cord index as a novel method of measuring cervical spine geometry to predict the chronic stinger syndrome in American football players. *J Neurosurg Spine.* 2009;11(3):264-271.

QUESTION 23

What Are Effective Clinical Techniques to Improve the Thoracic Spine Mobility Necessary for Shoulder Function?

Barton E. Anderson, MS, AT, ATC

An understanding of the need to treat the thoracic spine in patients suffering from shoulder pain and dysfunction has increased over the last several years. The thorax provides a structural base from which the scapula moves. There are multiple muscle attachments between the 2 structures. During overhead motions, such as throwing, the freestyle swim stroke, and the tennis serve, the thoracic spine is required to side bend, rotate, and extend to allow for appropriate scapular movement.[1] Consequently, a lack of thoracic spine mobility can negatively affect scapular and glenohumeral range of motion, muscle activation, and general shoulder function.

Mobility restrictions in the thoracic spine can be caused by a host of factors, including soft tissue adhesions, altered joint mechanics, muscle imbalances, poor spinal stability, and faulty movement patterns.[2] The wide variety of potential causes requires clinicians to consider a multifaceted approach to improving thoracic spine mobility. In choosing the best clinical techniques to improve thoracic spine

Huxel Bliven KC, ed. *Quick Questions in the Shoulder: Expert Advice in Sports Medicine* (pp 123-127).

mobility, clinicians must first appreciate the relationships between the thoracic spine and glenohumeral/scapular function and the possible causes for mobility restrictions.

Muscle imbalances, such as those identified in the Janda upper and lower crossed syndromes, can contribute to decreased thoracic spine mobility. Weakness of the deep cervical flexors, rhomboids, and lower trapezius muscles coupled with tight, overactive pectoralis major/minor, upper trapezius, and levator scapulae muscles produces the classic forward head and rounded shoulder posture.[2] This resulting posture leads to increased thoracic kyphosis. Overactivity of the rectus abdominis coupled with poor activation of the local spinal stabilizer musculature has also been suggested as a contributing factor for poor thoracic spine function. Finally, respiratory patterns of apical or chest breathing may also contribute to decreased thoracic mobility.[3] From these potential causes, it becomes necessary for the clinician to introduce multiple forms of intervention to improve thoracic spine mobility. Techniques to restore normal diaphragmatic breathing, lengthen and inhibit overactive musculature, activate weak musculature, and improve normal joint motion should be considered.

Restoration of normal respiratory patterns should be part of any rehabilitation program. It is especially important when trying to improve thoracic mobility. Good diaphragmatic breathing contributes to spinal stability by increasing intra-abdominal pressure and activating local spinal stabilizers.[2,4] Restoring diaphragmatic breathing patterns will also provide mobilization of the ribs and allow for greater mobilization of the thoracic spine.[3] Self-administered diaphragmatic breathing exercises can be implemented with patients as home care after proper instruction and cueing.[5] One such exercise involves the patient monitoring his or her breathing patterns with one hand placed on the abdomen and the other hand placed on the chest while in a supine hook-lying position (Figure 23-1). The patient breathes normally, focusing on inhaling and exhaling through the abdomen while keeping chest movement quiet.

Tight, overactive musculature can contribute to mobility restrictions and may be related to actual structural changes in the tissues or a neuromuscular response. A variety of soft tissue mobilization techniques, including instrument-assisted soft tissue mobilization, strain-counterstrain, massage, and others, can be used to inhibit and lengthen tight, overactive structures.

Following soft tissue mobilization, techniques can be used to increase thoracic extension and rotation, including movement exercises that target thoracic spine movement. Movements into thoracic extension and rotation help to re-establish normal articular mechanics, coordinate muscle activation patterns, and activate weakened and previously inactive muscles. Three commonly used exercises for improving thoracic spine mobility are presented here, but many others are available.

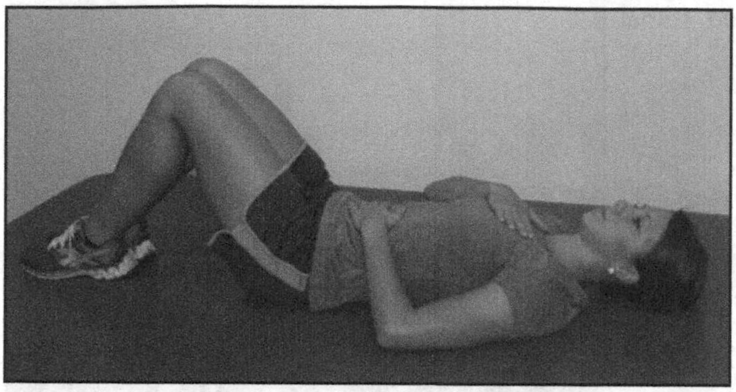
Figure 23-1. Hook-lying abdominal breathing.

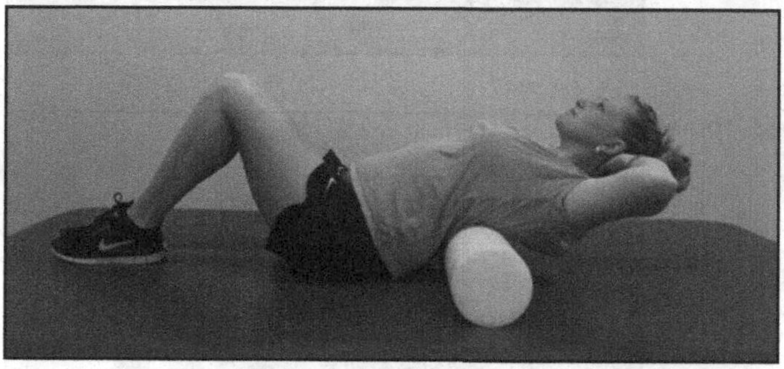
Figure 23-2. Thoracic extension on foam roller.

Thoracic Extension on Foam Roll

Thoracic extension improvements can be achieved using a foam roll placed perpendicular to the spine and having the patient slowly extend over the roll with his or her hands laced behind the head (Figure 23-2).[5] Focus should be placed on maintaining a stable lumbar curve during the movement and allowing the extension to come from the thoracic spine. Each extension can be held for 2 to 3 seconds, and the patient can work his or her way up and down the segments of thoracic spine.

Cat/Camel

From a quadruped position with the hands directly in front of the knees, the patient should arch his or her back as high as possible and then relax and slouch into spinal extension (Figures 23-3 and 23-4).[5] Focus should be on creating as much movement as possible and ensuring that cervical flexion and extension occur along with thoracic and lumbar movements. From quadruped, the exercise can be progressed by having the patient place his or her forearms on the floor or table with the elbows at the knees and repeat the arching/slouching movements.

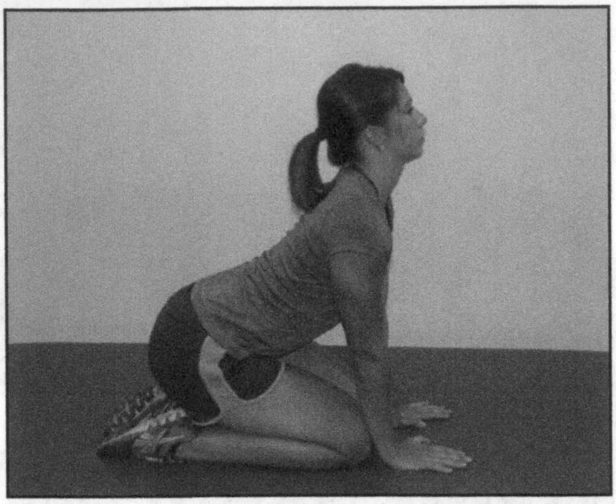

Figure 23-3. Reclined quadruped spinal extension ("cat").

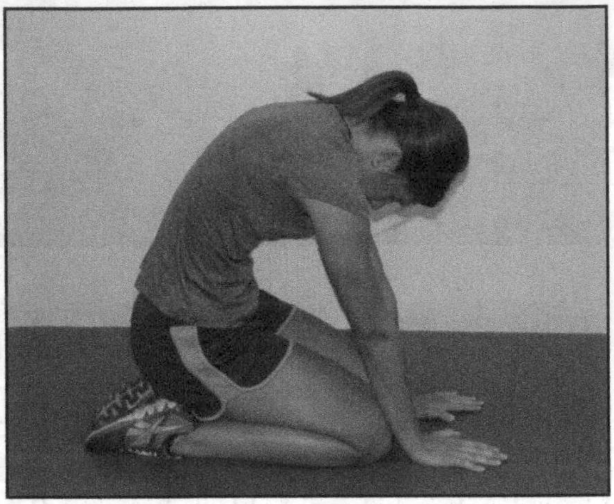

Figure 23-4. Reclined quadruped spinal flexion ("camel").

Quadruped Lumbar/Thoracic Rotations

From a quadruped position, the patient places one hand behind his or her head, lifts the elbow and head, and then rotates toward the same side (Figures 23-5 and 23-6). This movement will create rotation of both the lumbar and thoracic spine and will facilitate cervical, thoracic, and lumbar movements occurring in synchronization. The exercise can progress and the thoracic spine be isolated by having the patient rock back onto his or her heels, place the forearm on the table, and then repeat the rotation.

Thoracic spine mobility is a key component of normal shoulder function. Many different techniques exist for improving thoracic mobility, from manual joint manipulations and mobilizations to a variety of different movement exercises. Successful programs should be multifaceted and include interventions that target restoration of diaphragmatic breathing, normalization of muscle imbalance, and improvement of movement patterns in both extension and rotation.

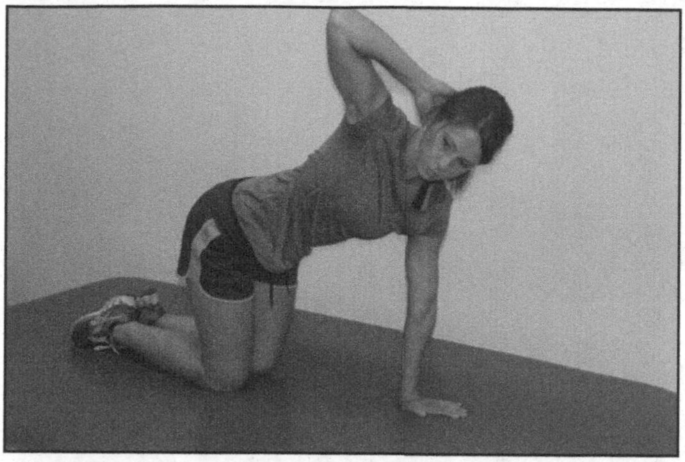

Figure 23-5. Quadruped rotation.

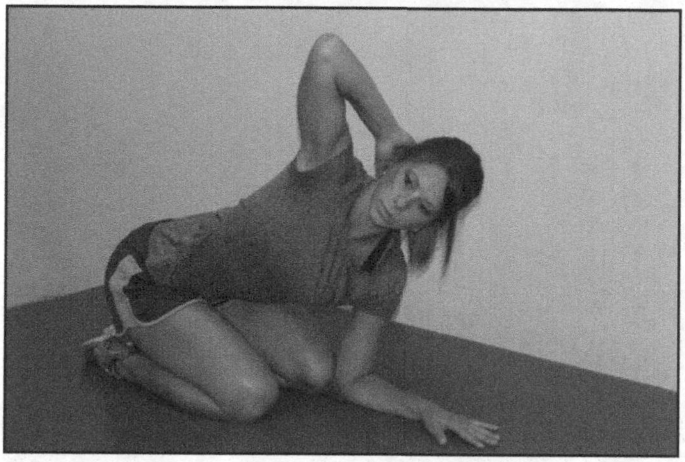

Figure 23-6. Isolated thoracic spine rotation.

References

1. Crosbie J, Kilbreath SL, Hollmann L, York S. Scapulohumeral rhythm and associated spinal motion. *Clin Biomech (Bristol, Avon)*. 2008;23(2):184-192.
2. Page P, Frank C, Lardner R. *Assessment and Treatment of Muscle Imbalance: The Janda Approach*. Champaign, IL: Human Kinetics; 2010.
3. Obayashi H, Urabe Y, Yamanaka Y, Okuma R. Effects of respiratory-muscle exercise on spinal curvature. *J Sport Rehabil*. 2012;21(1):63-68.
4. Huxel Bliven KC, Anderson BE. Core stability training for injury prevention. *Sports Health*. 2013;5(6):514-522.
5. Liebenson C. *Rehabilitation of the Spine: A Practitioner's Manual*. Baltimore, MD: Lippincott Williams & Wilkins; 2007.

QUESTION 24

What Are the Best Therapeutic Exercises for Addressing Scapular Dyskinesis?

Tim L. Uhl, PhD, ATC, PT, FNATA

Scapular dyskinesis is defined by either a static scapular malposition or dynamic alteration in scapular movement.[1] The scapulothoracic joint is not a true joint; it does not have a synovial lining but is dependent on and controlled by the surrounding muscles and joints. The scapulothoracic joint is critical for normal arm function because it works in harmony with the other true joints, the sternoclavicular, acromioclavicular, and glenohumeral joints, to provide the most mobile segment of the human body. The primary stabilizers and movers are called the axioscapular muscles and consist of the serratus anterior, all divisions of the trapezius, the rhomboids, the levator scapulae, and the pectoralis minor. The trapezius and serratus muscles have been found to be dysfunctional in the presence of pathology[2] and are conversely thought by some authors to be the cause of some shoulder pathologies. In either case, the prescription of exercises targeting scapular muscles is quite common.

The selection of exercises that target these scapular muscles is based primarily on electromyographic (EMG) research that has examined muscular activity during the

Huxel Bliven KC, ed. *Quick Questions in the Shoulder: Expert Advice in Sports Medicine* (pp 129-132).

performance of an exercise. Most of the research has been carried out on healthy individuals, which limits our interpretation of the results to cases of preventive intervention. However, there is growing evidence that exercises in patients with pathology (particularly with subacromial impingement) have decreased activation of the lower trapezius and increased activation of the upper trapezius. Evidence also shows that overall muscular activity is similar between healthy populations and patients with shoulder impingement.[3] Therefore, it is reasonable to take results on healthy subjects and apply them to an injured population, as long as one uses good clinical judgment in prescribing exercises at the appropriate level for a patient.

Exercises should be prescribed along a continuum from low- to higher-demand activities. Much of the literature has focused on high-demand exercises, but it is important to prescribe the appropriate exercise based on the patient's level of pain and dysfunction in order to have a positive effect. The best exercise is one that is performed correctly without aggravating symptoms, not the one that generates the most EMG activity. The clinician should consider prescribing exercises along a continuum to create the best intervention.

A review of shoulder exercises based on EMG evidence described several exercises that would form a core exercise program for addressing scapular dyskinesis.[4] Figure 24-1 was created by incorporating the exercises identified in the review but using the original authors' data plus those from one additional study that examined several scapular muscles during a push-up plus.[4,5] The exercises are organized in a progressive manner from low to high muscular activity and are primarily, but not exclusively, focused on lower trapezius and serratus anterior muscular EMG amplitudes. It is important to remember that muscles do not work in isolation. When available, all muscles are reported for the 3 portions of the trapezius and serratus anterior. Unfortunately, few studies have evaluated the rhomboids or the pectoralis minor, primarily because they are deeper muscles and require fine-wire needle insertion to measure muscle activity.

Muscular activity below 20% of maximal voluntary isometric contraction is considered low activity, 20% to 40% is moderate activity, 40% to 60% is high activity, and greater than 60% is very high activity.[6] The isometric low-row and inferior-glide exercises are low-demand exercises and de-emphasize the upper trapezius, which can be overly active in patients with rotator cuff impingement.[2] These 2 simple exercises are used to teach the patient scapular motor control because the patient would be working on retracting and depressing the scapula. As symptoms subside or in cases in which there is good motor control, exercises are progressed to more dynamic arm motions, such as wall slides, dynamic hug, lawnmower, and prone extension. These exercises can be selected based on individual needs to challenge either the lower trapezius or serratus anterior. Watch for substitution patterns and scapular dyskinesis while performing these exercises. If

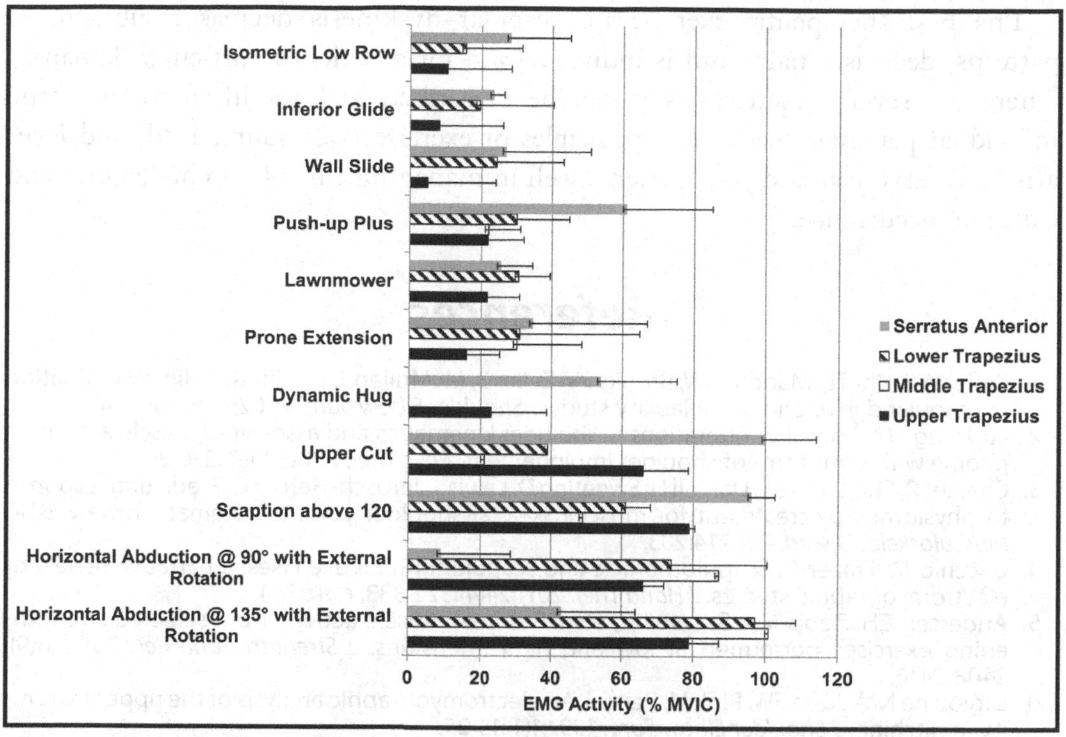

Figure 24-1. Scapular muscle exercise continuum. Abbreviations: EMG, electromyography; MVIC, maximum voluntary isometric contraction.

observed, make the exercises simpler by, for example, changing the lever arm or reducing the resistance. The push-up plus exercise is identified in this program but can be simplified by using a knee push-up plus or incline push-up plus. Lower loads reduce muscular demands. A wall push-up plus is often prescribed because it creates a lower load on the shoulder muscles, but it has been found to improperly increase upper trapezius activation over the serratus anterior, the targeted muscle during this type of exercise.[4]

The final 4 exercises are high to very high in muscular activation levels. The horizontal abduction exercises target the lower trapezius muscles, whereas the upper cut and scaption above 120 degrees exercises primarily challenge the serratus anterior. Prescriptions of these exercises are used to strengthen but should not be at the cost of creating substitution patterns with other muscles or aggravating a sore shoulder. When a patient has demonstrated a good foundation of scapular control with the lower-demand exercises, these higher-demand exercises can be introduced. In a healthy population, these exercises would be good candidates for use to prevent scapular dyskinesis. Increased loads and longer lever arms increase muscular demands during these exercises and can be modified to minimize substitution patterns.

The best therapeutic exercise for scapular dyskinesis decreases substitution patterns, decreases pain, and is individualized for a patient's particular demands. There are several exercises that can be prescribed and modified to meet the individual patient's needs. The principles of exercise continuum, load, and lever arm will serve you and your patients well in managing this often challenging and common occurrence.

References

1. Kibler WB, Uhl TL, Maddux JW, Brooks PV, Zeller B, McMullen J. Qualitative clinical evaluation of scapular dysfunction: a reliability study. *J Shoulder Elbow Surg*. 2002;11(6):550-556.
2. Ludewig PM, Cook TM. Alterations in shoulder kinematics and associated muscle activity in people with symptoms of shoulder impingement. *Phys Ther*. 2000;80(3):276-291.
3. Chester R, Shepstone L, Daniell H, Sweeting D, Lewis J, Jerosch-Herold C. Predicting response to physiotherapy treatment for musculoskeletal shoulder pain: a systematic review. *BMC Musculoskelet Disord*. 2013;14:203.
4. Cricchio M, Frazer C. Scapulothoracic and scapulohumeral exercises: a narrative review of electromyographic studies. *J Hand Ther*. 2011;24(4):322-333; quiz 334.
5. Andersen CH, Zebis MK, Saervoll C, et al. Scapular muscle activity from selected strengthening exercises performed at low and high intensities. *J Strength Cond Res*. 2012;26(9): 2408-2416.
6. Digiovine NM, Jobe FW, Pink M, Perry J. An electromyographic analysis of the upper extremity in pitching. *J Shoulder Elbow Surg*. 1992;1(1):15-25.

QUESTION 25

WHAT ARE THE MOST EFFECTIVE GLENOHUMERAL MOBILIZATION TECHNIQUES, AND WHEN ARE THEY MOST APPROPRIATE TO USE TO IMPROVE SHOULDER FUNCTION AND RANGE OF MOTION?

Bryce W. Gaunt, PT, SCS; Brian J. Phillips, PT, DPT; and Joseph H. Kostuch, PT, SCS

The glenohumeral joint is one of the most mobile joints in the body. Restrictions in range of motion (ROM) in any plane of movement can result in pathology and functional limitations. Joint mobilizations are often used in the painful or stiff shoulder to help improve ROM and function. When performing glenohumeral joint mobilizations, it is important for the rehabilitation provider to (1) have an accurate awareness of the glenoid fossa's orientation and recognize that it changes during elevation of the shoulder girdle, (2) mobilize primarily parallel to the glenoid fossa, (3) emphasize posterior-based mobilizations, and (4) assess and treat limitations at or near end ranges using low-load long-duration mobilizations. In addition, understanding when mobilizations are indicated and learning how to grade their dosage are important.

Contraindications to joint mobilizations include joint hypermobility and the presence of joint effusion, malignancy, and an unhealed fracture.[1] Indications for mobilizations include pain, muscle guarding, and reversible hypomobility

Huxel Bliven KC, ed. *Quick Questions in the Shoulder: Expert Advice in Sports Medicine* (pp 133-137).

and during periods of functional immobility.[1] It is not recommended to initiate glenohumeral mobilizations during the early postoperative period (first 6 weeks) after rotator cuff repair, capsulolabral repair, or shoulder arthroplasty. In addition, mobilizations after postoperative week 6 are recommended only if a patient's passive ROM (PROM) is behind targeted ROM goals.

Several well-known clinicians (eg, Kaltenborn, Maitland, Paris, and Mulligan) have described various mobilization techniques in the literature. Two popular mobilization strategies are graded oscillation and sustained translatory joint-play techniques.[1] Both strategies can be used for managing pain and as stretching maneuvers. Because the translatory joint-play technique is commonly used, it will be the focus of this chapter. Kaltenborn has described 3 grades of mobilization intensity. Grade I (loosen) mobilizations are small-amplitude distractions in which no stretch is placed on the capsule; these are mainly used to relieve pain.[1] Grade II (tighten) mobilizations apply enough force to "take up the slack" of the capsule up to tissue resistance but do not stretch the capsule.[1] They are used during primary assessment of joint mobility and also to help relieve pain. Grade III (stretch) mobilizations apply an amplitude large enough to stretch the joint capsule and surrounding periarticular structures.[1] These mobilizations attempt to stretch the joint structures to increase joint play.

An accurate awareness of the glenoid fossa's orientation is critical for glenohumeral mobilizations to be maximally effective. Accurate awareness of the glenoid's orientation is difficult because it cannot be directly palpated and because its position changes as the shoulder girdle moves. Winkel et al[2] described an indirect method for estimating the glenoid's position and orientation that can be used to guide glenohumeral mobilizations. They reported that in the frontal plane, the glenoid fossa is roughly perpendicular to the spine of the scapula (Figure 25-1), while in the transverse plane it is roughly parallel to a line connecting the posterior corner of the acromion with the lateral tip of the coracoid process (Figure 25-2). Finally, in the sagittal plane, the glenoid fossa is roughly perpendicular to a line connecting the posterior corner of the acromion with the lateral tip of the coracoid process (Figure 25-3). Considered together, these bony landmarks provide a composite picture of the glenoid's approximate position. They also help the clinician recognize that the orientation of the glenoid with the shoulder in 140 degrees of elevation is quite different, being more upwardly rotated, posteriorly tilted, and externally rotated than if the shoulder is positioned in 20 degrees of elevation. Accurate knowledge of the position of the glenoid with changing arm positions allows for accurate alignment and optimal application of the direction of force during mobilization.

Once the glenoid's position is established, it is fairly straightforward for the clinician to perform mobilizations parallel to the glenoid fossa. A posterior slide is

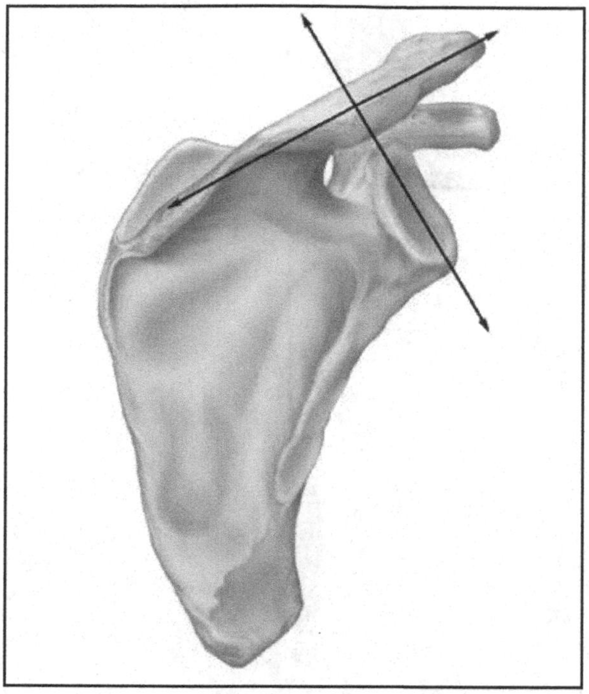

Figure 25-1. In the frontal plane, the glenoid fossa is roughly perpendicular to the spine of the scapula. This determines the amount of superior-to-inferior tilt of the glenoid. (Reprinted with permission from The St. Francis Orthopaedic Institute © 2014.)

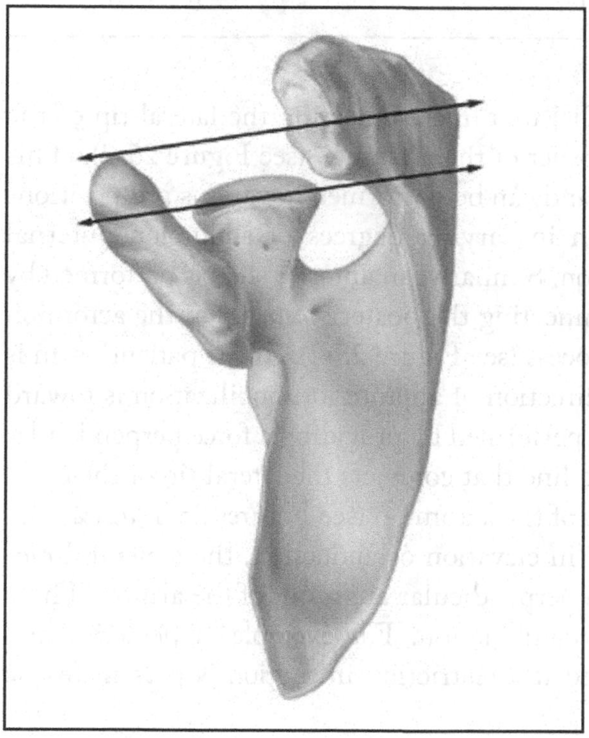

Figure 25-2. In the transverse plane, the glenoid fossa is roughly parallel to a line connecting the posterior corner of the acromion with the lateral tip of the coracoid process. This determines the anterior-to-posterior orientation of the glenoid. (Reprinted with permission from The St. Francis Orthopaedic Institute © 2014.)

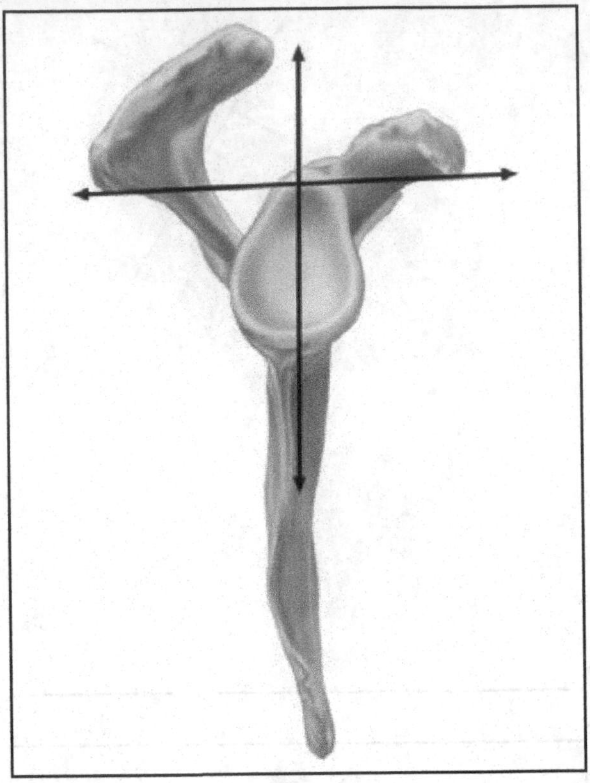

Figure 25-3. In the sagittal plane, the glenoid fossa is roughly perpendicular to a line connecting the posterior corner of the acromion with the lateral tip of the coracoid process. This determines the rotation of the glenoid. (Reprinted with permission from The St. Francis Orthopaedic Institute © 2014.)

performed by providing a force parallel to a line connecting the lateral tip of the coracoid process with the posterior corner of the acromion (see Figure 25-2).[2] This mobilization can be used extensively and can be performed in various pre-positions including elevation, external rotation in varying degrees of abduction, internal rotation, and even horizontal adduction. Similarly, an anterior slide is performed by providing a force parallel to a line connecting the posterior corner of the acromion with the lateral tip of the coracoid process (see Figure 25-2).[2] If the patient's arm is positioned in elevation, the general direction of an anterior mobilization is toward the patient's chin. An inferior slide is performed by providing a force perpendicular to both the spine of the scapula and a line that connects the lateral tip of the coracoid process with the posterior corner of the acromion (see Figures 25-1 and 25-3).[2] If the patient's arm is pre-positioned in elevation or abduction, the general direction of an inferior mobilization is at a perpendicular angle out of the armpit. These mobilizations can be performed in combination. For example, a posterior and inferior slide are commonly combined if a restriction in motion is present in the posterior inferior joint capsule.

Clinically, posterior-based mobilizations seem to be the most effective in many patients for improving not just limitations of PROM in internal rotation but also limitations of PROM in flexion, scaption, abduction, and even external rotation.

Using cadavers, Gerber et al[3] demonstrated that tightening the posterior capsule caused not only significant limitations in internal rotation ROM but also a 20-degree limitation in flexion and a 15-degree limitation in abduction. In a group of patients with adhesive capsulitis, posterior mobilizations in addition to a standard exercise program increased external rotation ROM an average of 31 degrees over 15 days, whereas anterior mobilizations and exercise increased external rotation ROM only 3 degrees over the same period of time.[4] These studies parallel clinical experience; when glenohumeral mobility is assessed carefully, the most common restriction is posterior, and posterior mobilizations seem to be the most effective at improving PROM in multiple planes of motion.

Besides having an accurate awareness of the glenoid's orientation, mobilizing primarily parallel to the glenoid, and emphasizing posterior-based mobilizations, the final component important for maximizing the effectiveness of glenohumeral mobilizations is to assess and treat at or near the end ranges using low-load long-duration mobilizations. Mobilizations primarily for pain relief are appropriately performed in mid-ranges of motion or in the loose-packed position. However, these positions are not ideal if the purpose of the mobilization is to increase PROM caused by adaptive shortening or contracture. In these instances, positioning the patient in a comfortable position at or near the end range of the restricted joint is necessary, so the mobilization can be done in an attempt to lengthen the abnormally shortened tissue. Restrictions in motion also seem to be very position specific, so the particular ROM restriction should be replicated as much as possible during positioning of the shoulder before beginning the specific joint mobilization. Long-duration holds are a primary component of almost all static muscle and joint-stretching programs. Although some recommend large-amplitude and/or high-velocity mobilizations to improve joint PROM, we prefer low-velocity, small-amplitude grade III mobilizations, because patients appear to have less muscle guarding and pain with this style of mobilization.

References

1. Kisner C, Colby LA. *Therapeutic Exercise: Foundations and Techniques*. 2nd ed. Philadelphia, PA: F.A. Davis; 1990.
2. Winkel D, Matthijs O, Phelps V. *Diagnosis and Treatment of the Upper Extremities: Nonoperative Orthopaedic Medicine and Manual Therapy*. Gaithersburg, MD: Aspen Publishers; 1997.
3. Gerber C, Werner CM, Macy JC, Jacob HA, Nyffeler RW. Effect of selective capsulorrhaphy on the passive range of motion of the glenohumeral joint. *J Bone Joint Surg Am*. 2003;85-A(1):48-55.
4. Johnson AJ, Godges JJ, Zimmerman GJ, Ounanian LL. The effect of anterior versus posterior glide joint mobilization on external rotation range of motion in patients with shoulder adhesive capsulitis. *J Orthop Sports Phys Ther*. 2007;37(3):88-99.

QUESTION 26

When Is It Best to Use Muscle Isolation and Muscle Integration Exercises in Shoulder Rehabilitation?

Michael T. McKenney, MS, AT, CSCS

Shoulder injuries are a common occurrence in many physical activities and sports. Subsequently, shoulders are often the target of rehabilitation programs prescribed by physicians, athletic trainers, and physical therapists. Two major goals of a rehabilitation program are pain reduction and improved function. Given the variety of strategies and techniques available, clinicians must engage in multifaceted decision making to accomplish these and other rehabilitation goals in an efficient and effective manner. The use of muscle isolation and muscle integration has a place and a purpose in shoulder rehabilitation. This chapter is intended to provide the clinician with an understanding of the appropriate use of both techniques.

Because the shoulder complex is composed of 3 bones, 4 joints, and more than a dozen muscles, it can be difficult to define and differentiate between isolated and integrated muscle-strengthening exercises for the shoulder complex. For example, if a patient performs an isolated exercise for abduction in which the deltoid is the prime mover, the scapular stabilizing muscles must fire simultaneously to maintain

Huxel Bliven KC, ed. *Quick Questions in the Shoulder: Expert Advice in Sports Medicine* (pp 139-141).

the position of the scapula on the thorax, and the rotator cuff must contract to ensure the integrity of the glenohumeral joint. Muscle integration refers to the multijoint, multiplanar, or co-contraction–producing movements. Examples of muscle integration exercises for the shoulder include the push-up, lat pull-down, and shoulder press exercises. In contrast, muscle isolation exercises refer to single-joint, single-plane exercises that target a specific muscle or muscle group. Isolation exercises involving the shoulder complex include the full-can exercise and scapular protraction exercises.

Traditional shoulder rehabilitation programs have typically included a period of rest and control of inflammation, followed by isolated and then integrated muscle strengthening. In developing the rehabilitation program, it is important to consider the strength demands and neuromuscular motor patterns specific to the physical activities or athletic skills performed by an individual.

Clinical experience and research results suggest that for a majority of shoulder rehabilitation cases, muscle integration is the most effective approach.[1] This recommendation is based on several factors. Muscles of the shoulder rarely, if ever, function in isolation. Voluntary movements of the upper extremity are controlled via motor programs that use coordinated groups of muscles and joint synergies, often in a proximal-to-distal fashion.[2]

Synergistic muscle control of the scapular muscles and rotator cuff plays an integral role in stabilizing the glenohumeral joint. This occurs when the glenohumeral joint is properly centered and optimal length tension is achieved in respect to the rotator cuff muscles. Complex movements (multiplanar, multijoint) and closed-kinetic-chain exercises provide an excellent practical approach to achieving this desired outcome. Axial loading of the humeral head in the glenoid fossa promotes co-contraction of stabilizing muscles, resulting in improved rotator cuff strength and joint stability.

Traditional thought led many clinicians to believe that isolated exercises were superior for restoring and improving muscle strength and hypertrophy of muscles during rehabilitation. However, clinical practice and recent research results show that multijoint exercises are equally as effective at producing strength gains and hypertrophy in the shoulder complex musculature.[3]

Isolated strengthening exercises in shoulder rehabilitation protocols must also be understood and used. During early phases of rehabilitation, it is often necessary to allow time for the body to heal and repair injured structures. This is an opportune time to take advantage of the benefits of muscle isolation and muscle strengthening exercises. Muscle isolation exercises can retard atrophy and promote strength and endurance without having a negative effect on injured tissues. The use of isolation exercises can be especially beneficial in setting the stage for intermediate and advanced integrated strengthening exercises. When using a corrective exercise approach, consideration should be given to initially targeting the underactive muscles in an effort to treat the cause of dysfunction.

The use of an isolated muscle approach should effectively transition to integrated muscle strengthening because it has been shown to be more effective at improving overall rotator cuff muscle performance.[4] Another time to consider isolated strengthening exercises is with patients presenting with specific neuropathy affecting individual muscles. Many studies have shown that individuals suffering with suprascapular nerve impingement can experience pain resolution and muscle bulk and strength improvement over a 6- to 12-month period with proper rehabilitation.[5] An important part of this rehabilitative prescription includes isolated strengthening exercises for the supraspinatus and infraspinatus. The purpose of this isolation is to restore the neuromuscular control of the specific muscles affected in an effort to reduce compensatory action from adjacent muscles (eg, posterior deltoid).

Conclusion

Both isolated and integrated methods of strengthening can and should be used in the rehabilitation of shoulder injuries. Improving strength and function must include consideration of the patient's status and the desired outcomes of rehabilitation. It must also include assessing and determining the need for and appropriate timing in the use of both isolated and integrated exercises.

References

1. McMullen J, Uhl TL. A kinetic chain approach for shoulder rehabilitation. *J Athl Train.* 2000;35(3):329-337.
2. Shumway-Cook A, Woollacott MH. *Theories of Motor Control: Theory and Practical Applications*. Baltimore, MD: Williams and Wilkins; 1995.
3. Gentil P, Soares SR, Pereira MC, et al. Effect of adding single-joint exercises to a multi-joint exercise resistance-training program on strength and hypertrophy in untrained subjects. *Appl Physiol Nutr Metab.* 2013;38(3):341-344.
4. Giannakopoulos K, Beneka A, Malliou P, Godolias G. Isolated vs. complex exercise in strengthening the rotator cuff muscle group. *J Strength Cond Res.* 2004;18(1):144-148.
5. Cummins CA, Messer TM, Nuber GW. Suprascapular nerve entrapment. *J Bone Joint Surg Am.* 2000;82(3):415-424.

QUESTION 27

What Are the Best Nonsurgical Treatment Approaches to Resolve Thoracic Outlet Syndrome and Improve Function?

Tim L. Uhl, PhD, ATC, PT, FNATA

Thoracic outlet syndrome (TOS) is a complex diagnosis that was addressed in Chapter 13. It is defined by compression of the neurovascular structures in the cervicobrachial region.[1] Nonsurgical treatment should focus on the following 4 primary areas: patient education, postural correction, muscular imbalance correction, and aerobic fitness.[1] Implementation of a multimodal approach has yielded positive benefits in 59% of patients with TOS.[2] A similar approach has been found to improve patients' self-report of disability that presented with both proximal and distal neurological symptoms.[3]

Patient education should focus on making the patient aware of provocative positions and strategies to avoid the positions that aggravate symptoms, such as sustained forward head posture or repetitive overhead motions. Sleeping and resting postures can also aggravate symptoms. Strategies to minimize stress on the cervical region include using a small towel to support the neck in neutral or a cervical pillow to minimize compression on the neurovascular bundle. Sustained posture should be avoided, particularly if sitting at a work station. There are several recommended

Huxel Bliven KC, ed. *Quick Questions in the Shoulder: Expert Advice in Sports Medicine* (pp 143-145).

postures for work stations and sleeping, and information about them is available on the Internet to educate patients.

Postural correction is important; however, addressing muscular imbalances is critical for ultimate recovery. Often, the rounded shoulder and forward head posture is present with TOS. The anterior pectoralis muscles are often tight, and the rhomboids and middle and lower trapezius muscles are lengthened and weakened.[4] In addition, the deep cervical flexors are weak, while the posterior suboccipital, upper trapezius, and levator scapulae muscles are short and tight. Addressing muscle imbalances by lengthening tissue should be done gently, often starting in support positions so that gravity does not overload the tissue. Most important in prescribing stretching exercises to a patient with neurological symptoms is that the symptoms need to be monitored so as not to irritate neurological tissues. In cases in which the tissues are easily inflamed, it is better to start with shorter periods of sustained holds, such as 5 or 10 seconds, and gradually increase them to 30 seconds. A popular stretch that is often prescribed is a corner stretch to lengthen the pectoralis muscles; however, great caution should be taken with this exercise, because patients often lean too far into the wall, which further loads the tight anterior tissues and can exacerbate the patient's symptoms. Although placing the arm in 90 degrees of abduction and 90 degrees of elbow flexion while horizontally abducting the arm lengthens the pectoralis minor, it can potentially overload the inflamed neurological tissue, so this stretch should be prescribed cautiously and may need to be modified based on the patient's symptoms.

Simultaneously working on strengthening the posterior scapular musculature, particularly targeting scapular retractors and cervical retraction, should be integrated into the treatment program to restore balance between the musculature. Initiating chin tucks, cervical extension, and scapular retraction in supported supine positions is a good starting point and is often tolerated because the neurovascular structures are not placed in a provocative position. Patients can be progressed from 5-second holds to 30-second holds while gradually increasing the number of repetitions performed. Deep cervical flexion exercises to increase motor control and endurance using biofeedback from a pneumatic stabilizer system can be incorporated to strengthen weak deep cervical flexors.[5] Progressing from isometric to isotonic exercises below shoulder level, such as low rows (shoulder extension with scapular retraction) and scapular retraction with shoulder external rotation, activates the lower trapezius, rhomboids, and posterior rotator cuff.[6] Those patients who have functional demands requiring overhead work or who are athletes should progress to doing shoulder-level or overhead exercises, such as prone horizontal abduction and prone horizontal abduction with arm abducted to 135 degrees; these are also called prone T and prone Y exercises, respectively. These exercises should be performed with full elbow extension and can place significant demands on cervical and shoulder musculature. Thus, these exercises should not be prescribed until the patient has mastered the lower-level exercises without an increase of symptoms.

The final component of the program is prescribing an aerobic exercise program to reduce pain and body mass. TOS symptoms are less likely to resolve in patients with a higher body mass index.[2] Aerobic exercise is important in weight management but also has been demonstrated to reduce symptoms in patients' chronic neck pain.[7] The American College of Sports Medicine recommends 150 minutes of moderate-intensity aerobic activity per week.[8] However, as little as 10 minutes 3 times per week is a good start, with gradual progression as tolerated by the patient and his or her symptoms. Before prescribing an aerobic program for a patient who is older, the patient may need medical clearance.

TOS is a challenging condition to treat; however, a multimodal approach has been found to have reasonable success. The key points in comprehensively treating TOS without surgery are educating patients on aggravating activities and postures, addressing muscle imbalance throughout the spine and upper extremity, correcting postural faults, and prescribing appropriate aerobic activities for those patients who are not already on an aerobic program to lose weight or to reduce stress on their nervous system. It is important to have physician clearance before the start of training to be sure that the patient is able to start an aerobic program.

References

1. Novak CB. Thoracic outlet syndrome. *Clin Plast Surg.* 2003;30(2):175-188.
2. Novak CB, Collins ED, Mackinnon SE. Outcome following conservative management of thoracic outlet syndrome. *J Hand Surg Am.* 1995;20(4):542-548.
3. Day JM, Willoughby J, Pitts DG, McCallum M, Foister R, Uhl TL. Outcomes following the conservative management of patients with non-radicular peripheral neuropathic pain. *J Hand Ther.* 2014;27(3):192-200.
4. Sahrmann SA. *Diagnosis and treatment of movement impairment syndromes.* St. Louis, MO: Mosby; 2002.
5. Jull GA, Falla D, Vicenzino B, Hodges PW. The effect of therapeutic exercise on activation of the deep cervical flexor muscles in people with chronic neck pain. *Man Ther.* 2009;14(6):696-701.
6. Watson LA, Pizzari T, Balster S. Thoracic outlet syndrome part 2: conservative management of thoracic outlet. *Man Ther.* 2010;15(4):305-314.
7. O'Riordan C, Clifford A, Van De Ven P, Nelson J. Chronic neck pain and exercise interventions: frequency, intensity, time, and type principle. *Arch Phys Med Rehabil.* 2014;95(4):770-783.
8. Chodzko-Zajko WJ, Proctor DN, Fiatarone Singh MA, et al. American College of Sports Medicine position stand. Exercise and physical activity for older adults. *Med Sci Sports Exerc.* 2009;41(7):1510-1530.

QUESTION 28

What Are the Most Important Range of Motion Restrictions After Shoulder Surgery?

Brian J. Phillips, PT, DPT; Bryce W. Gaunt, PT, SCS; and Joseph H. Kostuch, PT, SCS

After surgical repair of the shoulder (ie, acromioclavicular [AC] joint, rotator cuff, biceps tendon, labrum), the rehabilitation provider must have a thorough understanding of many factors related to the surgery to protect the tissues from deleterious effects. These factors include a detailed understanding of the surgical procedure, the general time frames of tissue healing, and the amount of stress applied to the healing tissues from specific rehabilitation exercises and activities.[1] The rehabilitation provider must always keep in mind that rehabilitation is only safe when the strength of the surgical repair or healing tissue is significantly greater than the stress that each exercise or intervention places on it. This requires knowledge of any passive range of motion (PROM) restrictions and the time frames of these restrictions, as well as knowledge of when it is safe to begin active range of motion (AROM) and strengthening exercises. The following information should be used as a general guideline for postoperative rehabilitation for the shoulder. There is considerable variability in surgeon preference on when to initiate the

Huxel Bliven KC, ed. *Quick Questions in the Shoulder: Expert Advice in Sports Medicine* (pp 147-152).

different phases of postoperative rehabilitation, and the rehabilitation provider is encouraged to consult the referring provider for the specifics of his or her preferred postoperative protocol.

Acromioclavicular Joint

AC joint injuries range from simple sprains to significant ligament and capsular tears with subsequent joint dislocation. When surgery is warranted, the extent of the surgical procedure will dictate the progression of postoperative rehabilitation (distal clavicle excision vs ligament reconstruction). After ligamentous reconstruction of the AC joint, AROM with the arm unsupported in an upright position should be delayed until biologic stability of the reconstructed tissue is established.[2] For an acute repair, this delay should be 4 to 6 weeks; for chronic repairs with significant soft tissue involvement, it may take up to 6 to 12 weeks.[2] The primary motions to avoid after any surgery to the AC joint are horizontal adduction of the shoulder (bringing the arm across the chest) and terminal elevation. It is recommended that the patient avoid passive horizontal adduction for 6 weeks and active horizontal adduction for 8 to 12 weeks to allow for adequate healing of any capsule or ligament resection or repair. Elevation restrictions may also be necessary after AC joint repair. Restrictions may include limiting passive elevation to 90 to 120 degrees, or even allowing no passive elevation for up to 6 weeks because of the significant movement at the AC joint during terminal shoulder elevation.

Rotator Cuff

Controversy exists about when to begin postoperative rehabilitation after rotator cuff repair. Early PROM exercises are recommended to minimize postoperative stiffness and limitations in range of motion (ROM).[3] Small- or medium-sized single-tendon repairs may require 6 to 9 weeks of strict PROM before beginning AROM or strengthening exercises. Large or multi-tendon massive repairs have a higher rate of re-tearing; therefore, surgeons may require at least 12 weeks of PROM to allow for adequate healing before beginning AROM or strengthening exercises.

Regardless of the size of the tear, certain planes of motion must be restricted to avoid straining the healing cuff. The primary planes of motion that should be restricted for both single and multi-tendon repairs include horizontal adduction and positions of functional internal rotation (IR) (Figure 28-1). These planes of motion are contraindicated during the first 6 weeks after surgery because they place

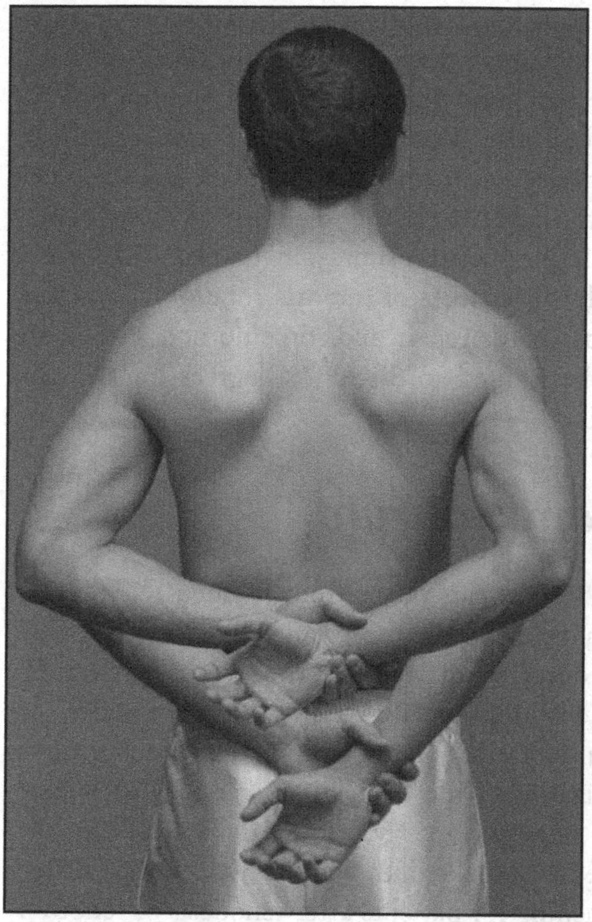

Figure 28-1. Active-assisted functional internal rotation stretch. (Reprinted with permission from Gaunt BW, McCluskey GM. *A Systematic Approach to Shoulder Rehabilitation.* Columbus, GA: Human Performance and Rehabilitation Centers, Inc; 2012.)

large amounts of strain on the repaired supraspinatus. This applies to PROM, active-assisted stretching, and AROM activities.

Abduction of the shoulder is cautioned during the entire rehabilitation process because of the high potential for impingement. Therefore, we recommend that overhead PROM, AROM, and strengthening be performed in the plane of the scapula to minimize impingement, improve scapular mechanics, and provide an optimal length-tension relationship to the rotator cuff, deltoid, and scapula muscles.

After rotator cuff repair, passive forward elevation in the plane of the scapula and passive external rotation (PER) at 20 to 30 degrees of abduction are recommended as the primary stretches during the first phase of rehabilitation. These motions place minimal stress on the supraspinatus tendon and seem safe to use during the immediate postoperative period.[3] These are the only 2 planes of motion in which patients need to perform PROM stretching at home during the first 6 postoperative weeks (POW).

Finally, care should be taken with passive external and internal rotation stretching at both neutral and 90 degrees of abduction during the first 6 POW. Cadaveric studies have shown that elevating the arm to 30 degrees of abduction prior to PER stretching helped reduce the tensile force placed on the cuff.[3] The authors demonstrated that external rotation up to 60 degrees in the scapular plane did not cause any significant increase in strain on the cuff.[3] A conflicting study[3] demonstrated a significant increase in strain to certain parts of the supraspinatus with a ROM of > 30 degrees of external rotation and > 30 degrees of internal rotation. Therefore, some surgeons limit PER after supraspinatus repair and some do not. If the subscapularis is repaired, PER should be limited to 30 to 45 degrees for the first 6 POW to protect the repaired tendon.

Biceps and Labrum

Surgeries that involve the biceps tendon can range from isolated tenodesis or tenotomy procedures to labral repairs involving the biceps anchor. These surgeries, especially the isolated biceps procedures, tend to have the greatest variability with postoperative rehabilitation. Rehabilitation after either biceps tenodesis or tenotomy has the same general consideration of allowing proper anchoring of the biceps tendon (via suture stabilization, bone anchor, or scarring) to prevent a popeye deformity. Some surgeons require no active elbow flexion for the first 4 to 6 POW. Consider waiting at least 6 weeks (although 12 weeks is preferred) before beginning any biceps strengthening for patients after tenodesis or tenotomy to minimize the risk of biceps cramping and potential popeye deformity.

After stabilization procedures for glenohumeral instability or superior labrum anterior-to-posterior (SLAP) lesions, patients should have a gradual, staged return of PROM targeting near-full PROM around postoperative month 3. It is important that the rate of ROM return be neither too quick nor too slow; a ROM table is often helpful to serve as a guide for ROM progression (Table 28-1).[4,5] For a patient with an anterior or multidirectional instability repair, the gradual return of external rotation, both near the side and at 90 degrees of abduction, is the most important direction to ensure sufficient shoulder stabilization.

SLAP lesions are commonly seen in baseball pitchers. In the late cocking phase of pitching, when the arm is placed in maximum abduction and external rotation, the biceps tendon winds upon itself, creating a peel-back mechanism that places a large shearing force on the superior labrum. This repetitive action is thought to be a contributing factor in SLAP lesions in pitchers.[1] Some surgeons restrict PER after a SLAP repair to minimize this peel-back stress. PER (at 20 to 30 degrees of abduction) may be restricted to 0 degrees of rotation for 3 weeks, progressing to 30 degrees during weeks 3 to 6, and finally to full ROM by weeks 6 to 8.[1] Full

Table 28-1

Postoperative Range of Motion Progression After Arthroscopic Capsulolabral Repair

Staged ROM Goals[a]

Postoperative Week	*Passive Forward Elevation*	*PER at 20 Degrees of Abduction*	*PER at 90 Degrees of Abduction*	*Active Forward Elevation*
1	100 degrees	10 to 30 degrees	Not applicable	Not applicable
3	130 degrees	20 to 40 degrees	Not applicable	Not applicable
6	150 degrees	45 to 55 degrees	45 degrees	115 degrees
9	165 degrees	50 to 65 degrees	75 degrees	145 degrees
12	Within normal limits	Within normal limits	Within normal limits	Within normal limits

[a]These are approximate targets for ROM. Specific limits might be specified by the physician. These ROM goals should not be greatly exceeded.

Reprinted with permission from Gaunt BW, McCluskey GM. *A Systematic Approach to Shoulder Rehabilitation*. Columbus, GA: Human Performance and Rehabilitation Centers, Inc; 2012.

PER ROM at 90 degrees of abduction should typically be achieved between weeks 8 to 12.

Special consideration is needed when the posterior aspect of the labrum is repaired. For this procedu
re, passive forward elevation stretching should be performed in the plane of the scapula, instead of sagittal plane flexion. The motions that are the most stressful to the posterior repair are horizontal adduction, functional IR, and IR in both adduction and abduction.[4] These motions are generally restricted until POW 6, and they are then gained in a progressive manner, targeting for full ROM at approximately POW 12.[4]

References

1. Dodson CC, Altchek DW. SLAP lesions: an update on recognition and treatment. *J Orthop Sports Phys Ther*. 2009;39(2):71-80
2. Mazzocca AD, Arciero RA, Bicos J. Evaluation and treatment of acromioclavicular joint injuries. *Am J Sports Med*. 2007;35(2):316-329.
3. Hatakeyama Y, Itoi E, Pradhan RL, Urayama M, Sato K. Effect of arm elevation and rotation on the strain in the repaired rotator cuff tendon. A cadaveric study. *Am J Sports Med*. 2001;29(6):788-794.
4. Gaunt BW. Arthroscopic capsular plication with or without Bankart repair. In: Gaunt BW, McCluskey GM, eds. *A Systematic Approach to Shoulder Rehabilitation*. Columbus, GA: Human Performance and Rehabilitation Centers; 2012:290-321.

5. Gaunt BW, Shaffer MA, Sauers EL, Michener LA, McCluskey GM, Thigpen C. The American Society of Shoulder and Elbow Therapists' consensus rehabilitation guideline for arthroscopic anterior capsulolabral repair of the shoulder. *J Orthop Sports Phys Ther.* 2010;40(3):155-168.

Question 29

What Are the Most Appropriate Exercises to Safely Gain Range of Motion Postoperatively With Minimal Activation of the Rotator Cuff Muscles?

Martin J. Kelley, PT, DPT, OCS and
Michael T. Piercey, PT, DPT, Cert. MDT, CMP, CSCS

Rehabilitation after shoulder surgery can pose multiple challenges for the sports medicine team. In particular, surgical procedures involving rotator cuff repair, tendon incision and repair (open Bankart), tendon relocation (biceps tenodesis), or osteotomy (shoulder arthroplasty and Latarjet procedure) can be somewhat difficult. The primary postoperative objective is to minimize the risk of excessive loads across the repair site. As such, in developing and implementing rehabilitation programs for these conditions, the clinician must consider a variety of factors. These factors include, but are not limited to, the need for immobilization (starting date, position, length of time), potential for development of postoperative stiffness, appropriate time for initiation of range of motion (ROM) exercises, and types of exercises that encourage motion without compromising the surgical repair. During the early postoperative phase, any of these factors can influence the rehabilitative course.

Huxel Bliven KC, ed. *Quick Questions in the Shoulder: Expert Advice in Sports Medicine* (pp 153-158).

A period of immobilization after shoulder surgery to protect the repaired tissue is common practice. Currently, the most common immobilization period after rotator cuff repair is 3 to 6 weeks. However, longer immobilization periods after rotator cuff repair have gained favor because multiple tendon-healing studies have shown that immobilization enhances tendon structure and strength and that Sharpey fibers do not appear until after 12 weeks.[1] Electromyographic (EMG) studies have demonstrated low muscular activation with specific shoulder ROM exercises,[2] as described later in this chapter, suggesting a decreased likelihood to result in re-tearing repaired tissue. Caution must still be practiced to further decrease this risk, especially when considering the re-tear rate that accompanies larger-sized repairs.[3] This may be accomplished by consulting with the physician to consider presurgery rotator cuff atrophy, tear location, size and quality of repaired tissue, surgical technique, past medical history, and risk for postoperative stiffness[4] because each of these factors will influence the immobilization period and exercises prescribed.

Although the initial period of immobilization appears to enhance healing, the development, or persistence, of stiffness can occur.[4] One systematic review indicated that it is common for patients to experience shoulder stiffness after arthroscopic rotator cuff repair, regardless of preoperative stiffness.[4] It is also important that the clinician be able to identify "appropriate" or "expected" stiffness after shoulder surgery. For example, 12 weeks after massive rotator cuff repair, a patient should still have limited external rotation (ER) with the arm at the side (about 30 to 40 degrees). The clinician should be mindful of this when working through any stiffness and attempting to increase motion. Despite experiencing some degree of stiffness, patients most often regain motion over time with conservative measures.[4] Arthroscopic capsular release may be required in patients who do not respond to conservative measures.[4,5] In a study completed by Huberty et al,[5] only 24 of 489 subjects (4.9%) experienced postoperative stiffness lasting more than 16 weeks after an initial arthroscopic rotator cuff repair.

As part of rehabilitation following rotator cuff repair, the clinician should initiate passive ROM exercises at 3 to 6 weeks. Typically, ER is restricted to 30 degrees. The ER motion should be performed with the arm on a pillow to avoid extension and at approximately 30 degrees of elevation in the plane of the scapula (POS; Figure 29-1). The exact timing and positioning should be dictated by the preferences of the surgeon. Some surgeons restrict elevation, whereas others do not. Passive motion is the goal, but clinicians should understand that EMG evaluation of shoulder musculature during passive exercises reveals some activity in healthy participants.[2] Supine forward elevation can be attempted, but it is often too painful because the patient cannot relax and the repair is being actively loaded. The clinician should palpate the deltoid to determine its activation; if active, he or she should assume that the rotator cuff is also active. The forward bow, or chair stretch,

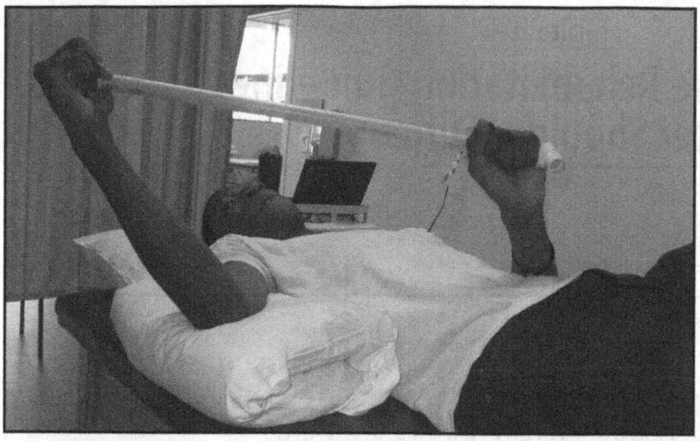

Figure 29-1. External rotation stretch to 30 degrees with the arm on a pillow.

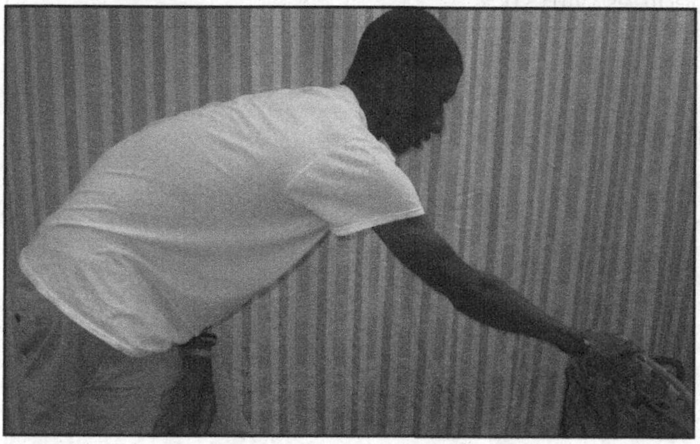

Figure 29-2. Forward bow (chair stretch).

exercise is often preferred, because it moves the body relative to the arm, has very low EMG activity, and is often much less painful (Figure 29-2). Typically, stretches are held for 10 seconds, because it is pain that is restricting motion rather than the connective tissue length. However, if true fibrosis is thought to be developing, the hold time should be increased toward 30 seconds.

Six weeks after surgery, increased gradual loading is appropriate. Regardless of the surgical procedure, the involved site still needs to be protected. An elevation progression program can be performed by using active-assistive exercises or supported assisted exercises, such as overhead pulley, stick-assisted forward elevation, ball roll, and towel slide (Table 29-1). These exercises each demonstrate low rotator cuff muscle EMG activation (less than 20% maximum voluntary contraction).[2] Both ROM and strengthening is achieved because the exercises incorporate partial weight of the extremity. The patient may start with supine stick overhead and progress to single arm raise. The surface can then be inclined so the weight of the extremity is increased (Figure 29-3). Standing ball roll below shoulder level can be progressed to rolling the ball on an inclined table and then up the wall

Table 29-1 **Early-Phase Rehabilitation Guidelines After Shoulder Surgery**

Day 1 to 4 to 6 weeks:
  Immobilization
  Active ROM of elbow, forearm, wrist, hand

3 to 6 weeks to 6 to 12 weeks:
  Passive ROM
    Chair stretch
    Supine forward elevation by uninvolved upper extremity
    ER stretch in POS to 30 degrees with stick

After 6 to 12 weeks:
  Active-assistive ROM
    Supine forward elevation with stick*
    Standing ball roll*
    Seated towel slide*
    Quadrant stretch (relaxing stretch)
    Overhead pulley*
    Standing extension
    Standing IR: hand behind back
    Horizontal adduction
  Active ROM
    Active supine forward elevation*
    Active supine forward elevation on inclined surface (gatching)*
    Standing ball roll on inclined surface*
    Standing ball roll up wall*

*Elevation progression.

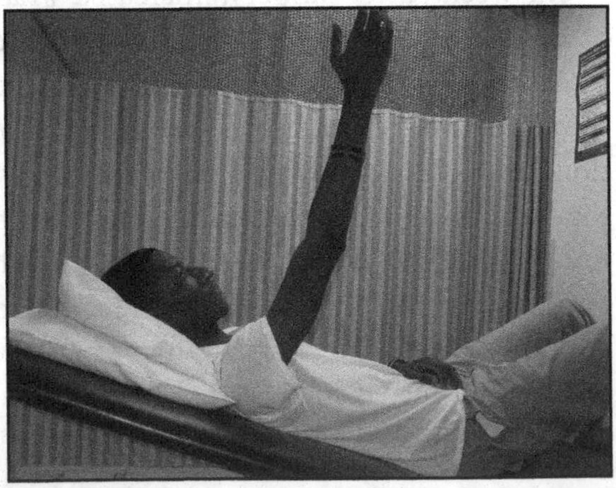

Figure 29-3. Supine forward elevation on an inclined surface.

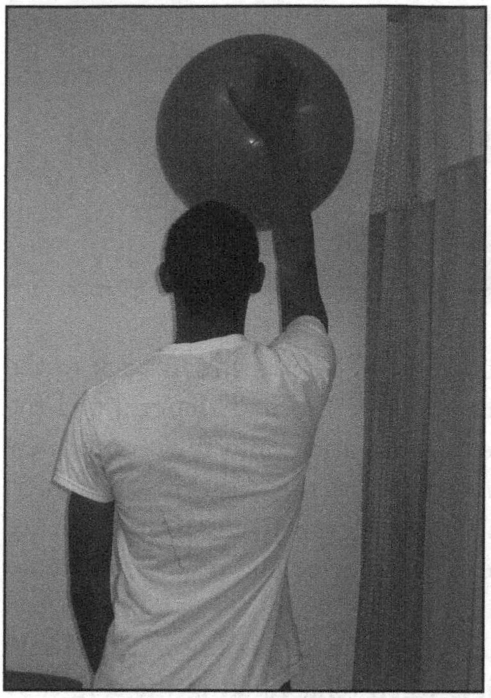

Figure 29-4. Standing ball roll up the wall.

(Figure 29-4). The pulley is a simple but effective device to use to regain elevation for either sustained stretch or active-assisted elevation. A nuance to using the pulley for motion is maintaining the elbow of the operated extremity in approximately 15 to 20 degrees of flexion when starting vs greater elbow flexion. If the patient has the elbow flexed to 90 degrees and the arm is pulled up, the shoulder must first externally rotate, twisting both the rotator cuff and capsuloligamentous complex. This action will limit greater elevation because the slack in the capsuloligamentous complex is already taken up and the consequence is usually pain. Another useful ROM exercise to regain ER at 90 degrees is to place the patient supine with the patient's hands resting (fingers locked) on an appropriate point on the head (forehead, top or back of head) with the elbows forward so that the patient is pain free. The elbows are gently dropped back to the point of slight pain by relaxing the pectoral muscles. This position is held for 10 to 15 seconds, and then the elbows are brought forward to relieve the pain (Figure 29-5).

During postsurgery weeks 6 to 12, active-assistive standing shoulder extension, internal rotation, and horizontal adduction can be initiated. The clinician needs to recognize that these exercises can place significant passive tension on the repair site. As such, the progression should be gradual. Patients who underwent a repair for a large or massive rotator cuff tear will typically begin these exercises after 12 weeks.

Another consideration for the clinician is the patient with a chronic, relatively asymptomatic supraspinatus tear with retraction who experiences an acute

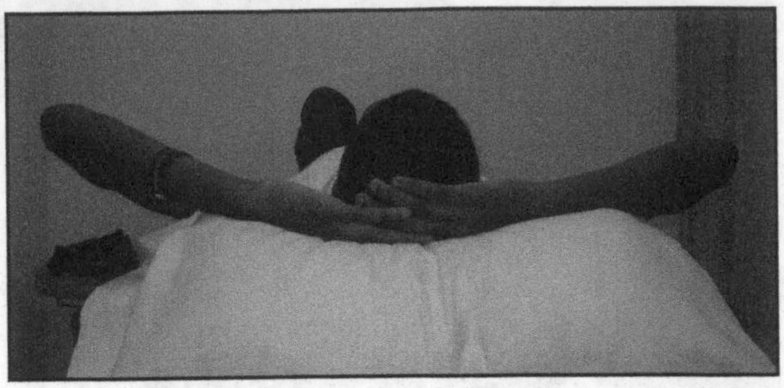

Figure 29-5. Supine external rotation stretch at 90 degrees.

infraspinatus tear. The surgery requires mobilizing the supraspinatus back to the boney insertion site. The muscle-tendon unit is not of "normal" length, and the potential excursion is limited. Stretching this type of patient into functional internal rotation (up the back) or horizontal adduction (across the chest) places significant tension on the supraspinatus and infraspinatus, respectively. Restrictions of internal rotation and horizontal adduction are to be expected and respected because of the nature of the repair.

A period of immobilization, paired with a gradual progression of ROM and low, controlled loading seems most appropriate when rehabilitating the surgically repaired shoulder to ensure optimal tissue healing. Although stiffness may occur, it is an acceptable complication that can be managed conservatively when compared with the possibility of re-tear. Implementing an elevation progression program by graduating through passive, active-assistive, and active motions allows the extremity to safely gain ROM.

References

1. Sonnabend DH, Howlett CR, Young AA. Histological evaluation of repair of the rotator cuff in a primate model. *J Bone Joint Surg Br.* 2010;92(4):586-594.
2. Uhl TL, Muir TA, Lawson L. Electromyographical assessment of passive, active assistive, and active shoulder rehabilitation exercises. *PM R.* 2010;2(2):132-141.
3. Bishop J, Klepps S, Lo IK, Bird J, Gladstone JN, Flatow EL. Cuff integrity after arthroscopic versus open rotator cuff repair: a prospective study. *J Shoulder Elbow Surg.* 2006;15(3): 290-299.
4. Denard PJ, Ladermann A, Burkhart SS. Prevention and management of stiffness after arthroscopic rotator cuff repair: systematic review and implications for rotator cuff healing. *Arthroscopy.* 2011;27(6):842-848.
5. Huberty DP, Schoolfield JD, Brady PC, Vadala AP, Arrigoni P, Burkhart SS. Incidence and treatment of postoperative stiffness following arthroscopic rotator cuff repair. *Arthroscopy.* 2009;25(8):880-890.

QUESTION 30

What Are the Most Important Aspects of Patient Education and Home Exercise Programs for Improving Shoulder Function?

Aaron Sciascia, MS, ATC, NASM-PES

Musculoskeletal rehabilitation is a dynamic process that is aimed at resolving identified physical impairments or injury. To address the deleterious effects of physical impairments and injury, multimodal treatment regimens are frequently employed and can produce promising results.[1,2] With many tools available to a clinician, the most common and possibly most important tools are patient education and home exercise programs (HEPs). Patient education involves informing the patient of the diagnosis, providing an expected prognosis and outcome, explaining the purpose of the exercises, and prescribing activity modification to avoid exacerbating current symptoms and to reduce or eliminate poor motor patterns. Most often, activity modification requires a review and modification of activities of daily living (ADL) and/or complex tasks such as manual labor or athletic maneuvers.

HEPs serve as part of a comprehensive rehabilitation program and are the physical component of patient education. Initially, basic maneuvers, such as single planar exercise and static stretching, are overseen by the clinician within the rehabilitation setting. Once mastered by the patient in the clinician's presence, the maneuvers

Huxel Bliven KC, ed. *Quick Questions in the Shoulder: Expert Advice in Sports Medicine* (pp 159-163).

are placed into a HEP. The goal is for patients to perform the foundational exercises away from the clinician so that more time can be spent on more challenging progressive exercises that require expert supervision. In addition, patients can enjoy personal achievement by mastering basic exercises, which in turn serves as a constant motivator for future therapeutic exercise progressions. HEPs complement formal supervised rehabilitation by influencing the motor system re-education process through daily exposure to and repetition of therapeutic exercise.

Patient education and HEP development should include purposeful therapeutic components designed to address each individual patient's needs rather than generic predetermined maneuvers. For example, not all patients present with identical symptoms with similar impairments and/or injury. As such, it would not be beneficial to a patient with mild impairments to perform rudimentary maneuvers, whereas the patient with more impairments and dysfunction would benefit from performing basic exercises. In either case, individual patient needs should guide the clinician and information provided to the patient. Similarly, patients who benefit from nonoperative treatment approaches will often be able to perform more advanced maneuvers earlier in the rehabilitation process than will postoperative patients, who require a more stringent level of protection to allow newly repaired tissue to heal adequately. Therefore, these considerations should be accounted for when developing patient education and HEP material.

In addition to individual patient needs, the complexity of the shoulder, in both anatomical composition and dynamic function, can create challenges for clinicians in providing appropriate patient education and in developing HEPs. To overcome the potential challenges, one method of patient education and HEP development specific to the shoulder is Bernstein's motor control theory. Bernstein theorized that there are many degrees of freedom or possible segment positions and motions from the foot to the hand during specified tasks.[3] This so-called redundancy is built into the human system to facilitate adjustment to both internal and external stimuli such as error feedback, fatigue, soreness, and/or environmental changes. A clinician's purpose in rehabilitation is to assist the patient in mastering the redundant degrees of freedom, which can be managed with patient education on proper movement patterns and HEPs designed for improving physiological function.

Initial patient education instructions should be managed through description and demonstration of how to perform arm-specific ADL. Patients should be encouraged to eliminate or at least reduce motions that exacerbate their current symptoms, which is most often accomplished through the restriction of long-lever arm movements, such as performing tasks at or above 90 degrees of forward elevation and/or abduction. If the maneuvers cannot be eliminated because of daily life requirements, the tasks can be modified in either of 2 manners. First, the arm position can be modified to a short-lever position, with the arms at the side of the body and

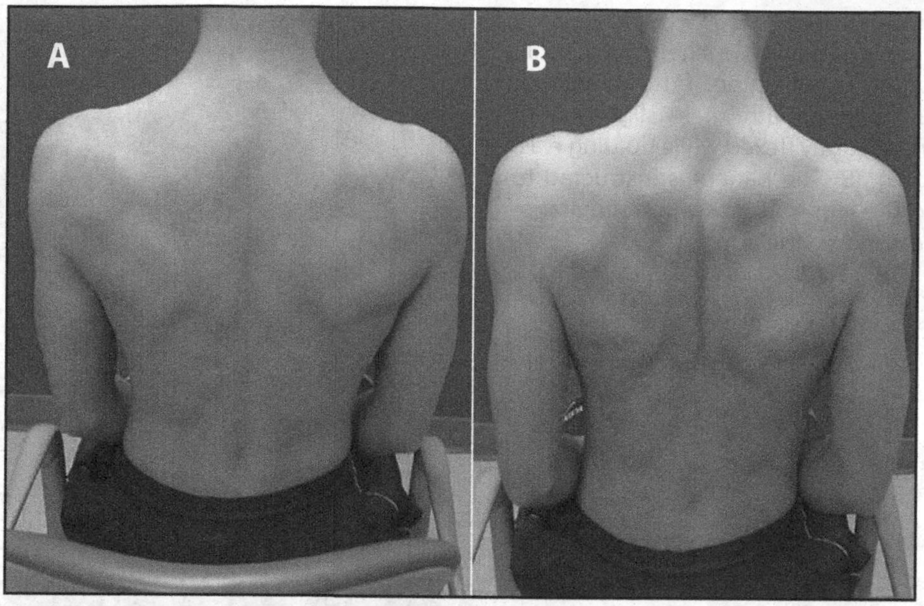

Figure 30-1. Focal scapular positioning in a seated position aims to achieve foundational muscle re-education by limiting the degrees of freedom from other body segments. (A) The patient should begin seated with the arms in a resting position and then (B) actively retract the scapulae without shrugging the shoulders or extending the spine.

elbows flexed to 90 degrees. This modification can allow a person to perform tasks in front of the body while reducing the stress placed on the shoulder. The alternative modification is to encourage patients to reduce the stress on the shoulder by using the larger kinetic-chain segments (ie, the legs and trunk) during arm-specific tasks. This is best illustrated with an example of reaching to a high shelf. It is common for individuals to stand with both feet securely on the floor and with a rigid trunk when reaching above shoulder height to place or retrieve an item from a high shelf. To accentuate both the stability and movement function of the lower extremity and trunk during overhead reaching, patients should be directed to shift their weight toward the task by extending the legs and trunk. If patients are unable to perform this modification adequately, a step or other assistive device can be used, which would also shorten the arm lever during overhead reaching. Clinicians should routinely assess patient ADL task execution and provide external feedback, which will assist in improving motor control.

Exercises to be contained within an HEP should begin with maneuvers that reduce or constrain redundant motions. For example, optimal scapular motion should be achieved in the initial phases of shoulder rehabilitation.[4] Clinicians can help patients reduce excessive body motions by having them perform scapular positioning exercises in a seated position (Figure 30-1). The seated position minimizes the number of body segments the patient can use by restricting the use of the lower

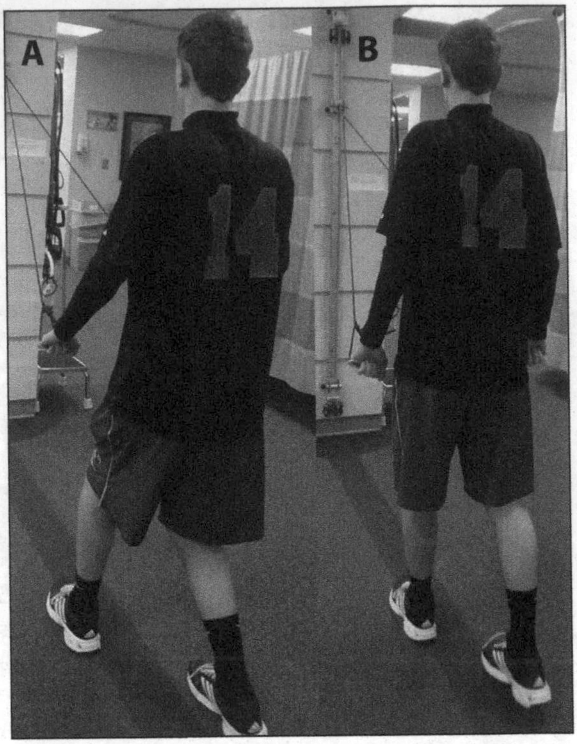

Figure 30-2. The low row exercise uses integrated trunk and hip extension to facilitate scapular retraction. (A) The patient begins standing with knees slightly bent and arms slightly flexed while holding elastic tubing. (B) The patient is instructed to extend the legs and hips while simultaneously extending the arms.

extremity segments. The patient can then be allowed to stand upright, bringing in the pelvic girdle and lower extremity influences on the trunk. These lower segments also have a significant influence on scapular motion because they so greatly affect trunk function. The HEP should follow a chain of difficulty from fewer to greater influences affecting scapulohumeral motion. Once the constrained movements have been mastered, the patient can then be allowed to use more anatomical segments to facilitate larger movements, such as trunk and hip extension to facilitate scapular retraction (Figure 30-2).[4,5]

Patient compliance is a routine concern of practicing clinicians, so effort must be expended to ensure that patients adhere to their HEP. To increase compliance, a HEP should start with proximal influences and progress to more distal kinetic-chain influences. They should be reasonable in length (no more than 3 to 5 exercises or stretches) and should contain foundational maneuvers that can be performed safely by the patient without direct oversight by a clinician. In addition, HEP performance should be tracked for compliance with daily logs. Clinicians should periodically review the HEP for content and discuss any concerns the patient may have regarding the performance of any of the exercises within the program. These efforts can enhance the patient-clinician relationship and improve HEP compliance.

References

1. Holmes CF, Fletcher JP, Blaschak MJ, Schenck RC. Management of shoulder dysfunction with an alternative model of orthopaedic physical therapy intervention: a case report. *J Orthop Sports Phys Ther.* 1997;26(6):347-354.
2. Tate AR, McClure PW, Young IA, Salvatori R, Michener LA. Comprehensive impairment-based exercise and manual therapy intervention for patients with subacromial impingement syndrome: a case series. *J Orthop Sports Phys Ther.* 2010;40(8):474-493.
3. Sporns O, Edelman GM. Solving Bernstein's problem: a proposal for the development of coordinated movement by selection. *Child Dev.* 1993;64(4):960-981.
4. Sciascia A, Cromwell R. Kinetic chain rehabilitation: a theoretical framework. *Rehabil Res Pract.* 2012;2012:853037.
5. McMullen J, Uhl TL. A kinetic chain approach for shoulder rehabilitation. *J Athl Train.* 2000;35(3):329-337.

SECTION IV

THE OVERHEAD ATHLETE

QUESTION 31

What Assessments Should Be Used in Screening Overhead Athletes to Determine Increased Risk for Injury? If Screening Indicates Injury Risk, What Injury Prevention Strategies Are Recommended?

Ellen Shanley, PhD, PT, OCS

Overhead athletes play sports that rely on the efficient replication of functional movement. The patterns of movement impart mechanical forces that affect the athlete's soft tissue and bone and are manifested as asymmetrical range of motion (ROM), flexibility, and imbalances in muscle performance. The development of injury is believed to be multifactorial and include physical and performance factors that are related to the sport and position played by the athlete. It is helpful to establish athlete-specific musculoskeletal baselines to enable changes in these factors to be identified and corrected before the manifestation of injury.

The American College of Sports Medicine has advocated screening at the preparticipation physical to identify at-risk athletes and to develop strategies to prevent injury.[1] These preparticipation screenings are often general and work well for athletes without a history of injury and those participating in multiple sports.

Huxel Bliven KC, ed. *Quick Questions in the Shoulder: Expert Advice in Sports Medicine* (pp 167-171).

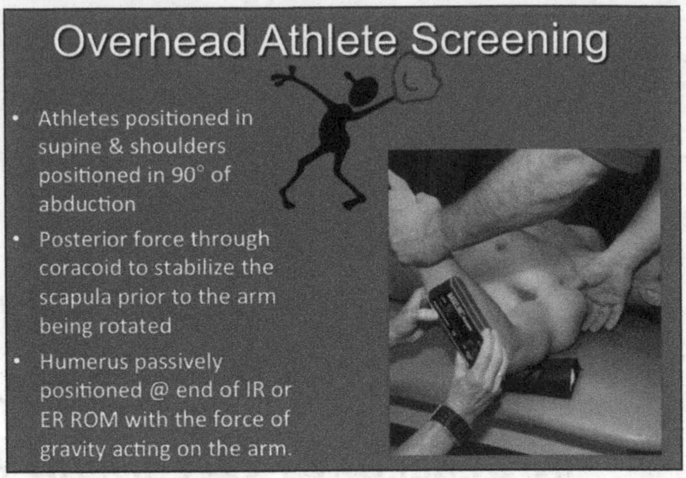
Overhead Athlete Screening
Athletes positioned in supine & shoulders positioned in 90° of abduction
Posterior force through coracoid to stabilize the scapula prior to the arm being rotated
Humerus passively positioned @ end of IR or ER ROM with the force of gravity acting on the arm.

Figure 31-1. Sample training slide showing measurement of shoulder rotation. (Reprinted with permission from Ellen Shanley, PhD, PT, OCS, CSCS.)

However, additional sport-specific screening may be beneficial for competitors consistently focusing on one sport or position and those with a history of injury. For the overhead athlete, screening should focus on identifying the athletes susceptible to injury based on known risk factors, including previous injury history, excess exposure (ie, pitch counts or rest periods), rapid periods of physical growth, deficits or imbalances in ROM and strength, and asymmetrical kinetic-chain performance.[2] Longitudinal screening that includes a minimum of 2 time points (pre- and post-season) per uninjured athlete is recommended.

The most efficient screening involves staggering athletes from the same team to progress through several checkpoints during a given session before the start of a practice. It is recommended that use of a training power point and practice session with all clinicians involved in the screening process be adopted to ensure familiarity with and reliability of the techniques, paperwork, procedures, and equipment used before execution of the screening (Figure 31-1).

Items for screening depend on many factors, including the type of athletes and level of participation (ie, youth baseball vs collegiate swimming), resources and time available for screening, and the needs and support of the community. The minimum screening recommendations for facilities with limitations in equipment or personnel are 2 stations. The first station documents general demographics (height, weight, hand dominance, position played, number of teams played per year, and previous injuries), and the second screening station examines functional movements (ie, overhead squat with arms fully elevated) to expose limitations in segmental flexibility and neuromuscular control. Additional screening stations require equipment to monitor joint-specific function that may not be routinely available (eg, a treatment table and goniometer to examine shoulder ROM in the overhead athlete). This basic level of screening may not identify specific impairments that require attention, but it helps to identify athletes requiring more complete evaluation and to target the follow-up examination.

Ideally, a more complete screening would incorporate the most commonly identified modifiable risk factors from the literature. The risk factors that have been associated with injury in youth and adolescent athletes in prospective studies include ROM and strength and are prioritized for screening. Other risk factors cited in retrospective studies or hypothesized based on similar populations are included secondarily, such as Beighton score, humeral torsion, and lower extremity balance. Therefore, the preferred screening system includes both segmental upper extremity and whole-body screening. Screening may begin with collecting baseline height, weight, hand dominance, positions of play, Beighton score, previous exposure, and the athlete's subjective assessment of discomfort and current function. The second station may involve assessment of bilateral ROM for the glenohumeral joint (external rotation/internal rotation and horizontal adduction) and elbow joint (elbow extension in neutral and fully supinated positions). Ultrasonography may be used to measure bilateral humeral torsion. Baseline strength and then endurance for the glenohumeral joint (external rotation/internal rotation and full can position-strength; prone horizontal adduction for endurance) are assessed after the ROM assessment. The athlete can then proceed to the functional assessment station, testing overhead squat, scapular dyskinesis, prone plank, and Y balance. The results of the screening are documented to enable the communication of results and tracking of impairments and to form the basis of our prevention programs.

Although a prevention program individualized to each athlete's impairments would be optimal, the practical management of athletic populations makes it unrealistic. A general pre- and in-season program (Figure 31-2) is recommended for all athletes who present with minimal impairments and low risk of injury after their most recent screening. For athletes with a history of injury or those demonstrating impairments that might elevate their injury risk, aggregating impairments into broader categories (eg, posterior flexibility) and prioritizing them within the context of their participation in the general program, as appropriate, are recommended. For athletes demonstrating multiple impairments or an injury history plus impairments, an individualized program specific to impairments that is closely supervised and progressed to minimize risk while enhancing performance is recommended. The athlete may be allowed to participate in the beneficial portions of the general conditioning program as long as participation does not increase his or her risk of injury or reinforce current impairments (ie, faulty movement patterns).

Additional screenings should be conducted for athletes presenting with discomfort, youth and early adolescents undergoing large growth spurts, athletes with a history of overuse arm injuries, and those presenting with impairments on the previous screen. Athletes should be screened regularly to ensure compliance and

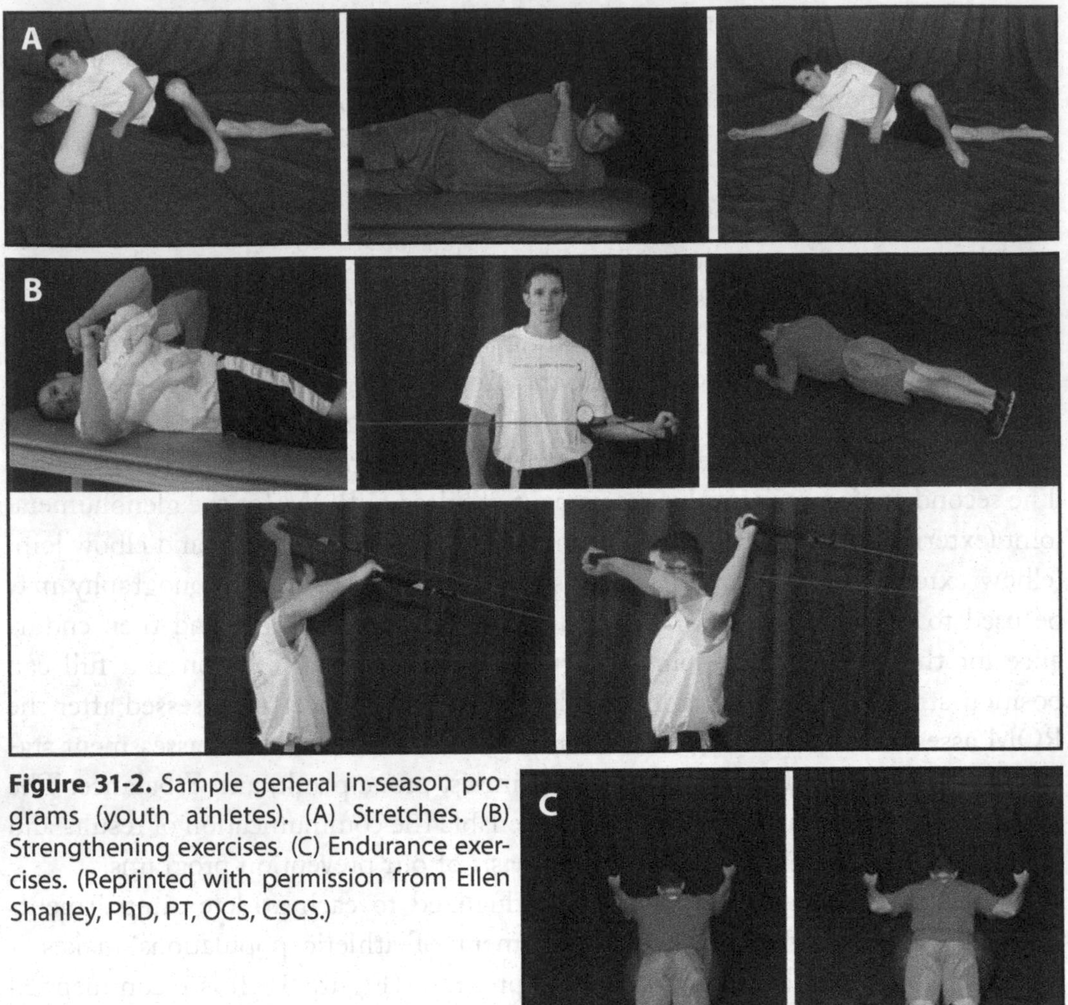

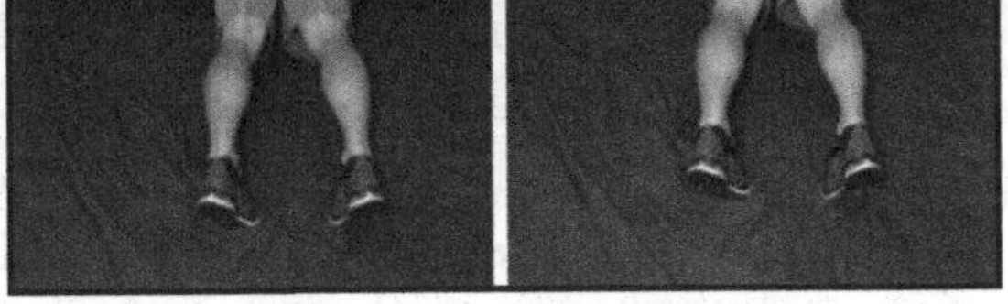

Figure 31-2. Sample general in-season programs (youth athletes). (A) Stretches. (B) Strengthening exercises. (C) Endurance exercises. (Reprinted with permission from Ellen Shanley, PhD, PT, OCS, CSCS.)

progress toward minimizing their deficits. Clinicians should track their athletes for the development of injury and reassess all athletes who report a time-loss injury. Reassessment involves the use of a functional outcome assessment and repeat screening with the appropriate tests based on athlete presentation and irritability. Screening of these athletes may be done in collaboration with their sport and health care team to maximize efficiency and minimize potential for exacerbation of their problem. Ideally, all athletes should receive a postseason screen, and the results of these screens should be combined with injury information to evaluate and modify the prevention program to maximize benefit.[3]

Conclusion

The most effective screening and injury-prevention programs are the efforts built on an understanding of the injury problem within the particular community, the identification and longitudinal tracking of risk factors, and implementation and evaluation of the results of prevention programs. The prevention efforts are cyclical and involve continual adjustments to the program.

References

1. Current comment from the American College of Sports Medicine. August 1993—"The prevention of sport injuries of children and adolescents." *Med Sci Sports Exerc.* 1993;25(8 Suppl): 1-7.
2. Valovich McLeod TC, Decoster LC, Loud KJ, et al. National Athletic Trainers' Association position statement: prevention of pediatric overuse injuries. *J Athl Train.* 2011;46(2):206-220.
3. Bahr R, Krosshaug T. Understanding injury mechanisms: a key component of preventing injuries in sport. *Br J Sports Med.* 2005;39(6):324-329.

QUESTION 32

Why Is It Important to Assess Shoulder Rotational Range of Motion in Overhead Athletes?

Kelsey Picha, MS, ATC and Eric L. Sauers, PhD, ATC, FNATA

Shoulder and elbow pain are common complaints among overhead athletes, particularly in throwing sports such as baseball. In youth baseball athletes alone, aged 9 to 14 years, more than 50% of pitchers suffer from pain in either joint.[1] Many factors may contribute to shoulder pain in overhead athletes; therefore, a thorough physical assessment is necessary. A key element of the shoulder examination is the assessment of upper extremity rotational range of motion (ROM). Overhead athletes need to have adequate ROM to enable movements into positions required for their sport, but they also require adequate stabilization to this highly mobile joint. Adaptations in shoulder ROM in overhead athletes are most widely reported in throwers, who sustain a significant number of shoulder injuries. Therefore, this chapter will focus on the overhead throwing athletes.

The stresses created during the throwing motion can alter the glenohumeral joint capsule, ligaments, and labrum as well as the articular and osseous structures. Repetitive overhead throwing may result in a tight or thickened posterior glenohumeral joint capsule, stiff musculature, and increased humeral retroversion.[2]

Huxel Bliven KC, ed. *Quick Questions in the Shoulder: Expert Advice in Sports Medicine* (pp 173-176).

Subsequently, a thrower may also experience alterations in shoulder rotational ROM because of the structural changes that exist from the repetitive trauma. Currently, some changes in rotational ROM are thought to result from adaptations to overhead throwing and may actually be protective and/or performance enhancing, whereas other ROM changes are associated with the development of shoulder and elbow injury. Clinicians should measure and attempt to differentiate how a throwing athlete's shoulder rotational ROM profile is affected by bony and soft tissue structural changes.

The shoulder should have approximately 0 to 90 degrees of internal rotation (IR) and 0 to 100 degrees of external rotation (ER) when measured at 90 degrees of abduction. However, studies have shown wide variability in what is considered normal for rotational ROM at the shoulder. Further, these numbers may differ significantly according to measurement technique (scapula stabilized) and in the presence of pain or muscle guarding. Throwers may have a difficult time relaxing during ROM measurements, especially of their dominant arm. It is important that the clinician demonstrate confidence to the patient and gain the patient's trust in holding and protecting his or her shoulder during the measurements, especially when injury-related pain is present. Practice is required to develop the appropriate technique to obtain precise and reliable measures of shoulder rotational ROM.

Every upper extremity examination of overhead throwing athletes should include an assessment of isolated glenohumeral (ie, scapula-stabilized) IR, ER, and total arc of rotational ROM (IR + ER) at 90 degrees of abduction (Figure 32-1). Both IR and ER at 90 degrees of abduction should be measured and recorded separately and then added together to obtain the total arc of rotational motion on both the throwing and nonthrowing shoulders.[2] Unidirectional IR and ER should be compared bilaterally for symmetry. However, it is quite common for individuals, especially overhead athletes, to have asymmetric shoulder rotational ROM. For instance, it is common for the throwing shoulder to exhibit greater ER with a concomitantly lesser degree of IR compared with those of the nonthrowing shoulder. This is most likely caused by osseous changes at the proximal humeral physis resulting from the extreme torque placed on the proximal humerus during the late cocking phase of throwing. Subsequently, a shear stress is created that prevents the normal age-related loss of humeral retroversion that should occur during maturation until the physis closes at around age 19 years. Changes in humeral retroversion should alter the throwing shoulder rotational ROM in a symmetric manner. That is, for every 1 degree of external rotation gained, 1 degree of internal rotation would be lost, because the shoulder is "spinning" backward at the proximal humerus. Subsequently, the shoulder is neither gaining nor losing total rotational ROM, and this combined motion should be equivalent to the total rotational ROM on the nondominant side.[2] Unless the athlete has a painful proximal humeral physis (eg,

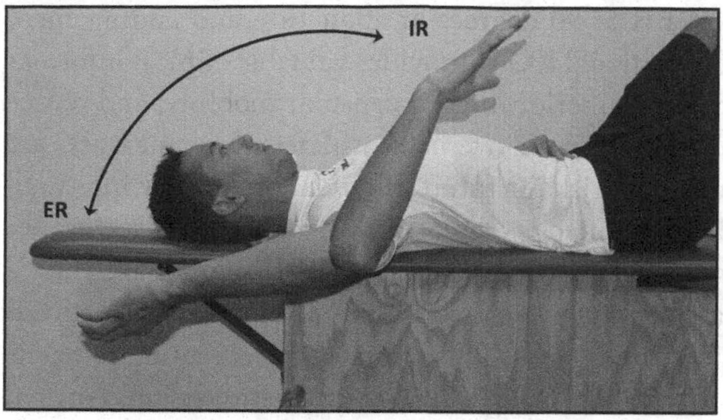

Figure 32-1. Glenohumeral rotational range of motion. Total arc of motion = internal rotation + external rotation.

Little League shoulder), this shift resulting in a symmetric total arc of rotational ROM is considered a normal osseous adaptation to the repetitive demands of overhead throwing.

If the total arc of rotational ROM is asymmetric, either larger or smaller, by greater than 10 degrees, the athlete may be at risk for shoulder and/or elbow injury. If the total arc of rotational ROM is larger by greater than 10 degrees, both IR and ER should be examined to determine from where the extra motion is coming. In most overhead throwers, a greater total arc of rotational ROM will result from greater ER in the throwing shoulder. Although some degree of increase in ER is considered normal for overhead athletes because of increased humeral retroversion, too much motion may be indicative of anterior-inferior capsulolabral attenuation and glenohumeral instability. Therefore, any overhead thrower with a total arc of rotational ROM that is ≥ 10 degrees more than the nonthrowing shoulder should be considered at risk for developing shoulder instability.[3]

Conversely, if the throwing shoulder's total arc of rotational ROM is ≥ 10 degrees less than the nonthrowing shoulder, risk for glenohumeral IR deficit (GIRD) should be considered.[4] Once again, although some loss of IR is to be expected because of changes at the proximal humeral physis resulting in greater humeral retroversion, too much loss of IR can be problematic. Although reports vary regarding the magnitude of GIRD that should be considered problematic, it is generally accepted that a loss of 20 degrees or more of IR is associated with both shoulder and elbow injury in overhead athletes.[5] Excessive loss of IR on the throwing shoulder is attributed to posterior glenohumeral joint capsule and rotator cuff scarring and contracture resulting in posterior shoulder tightness. Posterior shoulder tightness has been associated with altered scapular and humeral kinematics contributing to shoulder impingement and labral injury as well as ulnar collateral ligament injury in throwers.

The throwing shoulder is complex and can present a significant diagnostic challenge. However, a simple bilateral assessment of shoulder rotational ROM consisting of measuring IR and ER at 90 degrees of abduction and adding them together to asses the total arc of rotational ROM provides valuable clinical information regarding humeral retroversion, anterior-inferior capsular mobility, and posterior shoulder tightness. In healthy noninjured overhead athletes, these measures are a valuable screening tool for assessing risk for future shoulder and elbow injury. In patients with shoulder and elbow pathology, these measures are fundamental for assessing injury etiology. A healthy throwing shoulder will likely demonstrate a modest increase in ER with a concomitant loss of IR but a total arc of rotational ROM that is symmetric to within 10 degrees. This is a normal adaptation to repetitive overhead stress and is attributed to changes in humeral retroversion. Normal osseous changes will alter ER and IR but should result in a symmetric bilateral total arc of rotational ROM. A larger total arc of rotational ROM on the throwing side resulting from a significant increase in ER should alert the clinician to screen further for the presence of anterior-inferior instability and secondary impingement syndrome and/or internal impingement. A smaller total arc of rotational ROM on the throwing side resulting from a significant loss of IR should alert the clinician to screen further for the presence of GIRD and subsequent labral pathology and/or internal impingement. The clinical importance of assessing bilateral IR, ER, and total arc of rotational ROM cannot be overstated, given the wealth of information that can be deduced regarding potential osseous and soft tissue changes at the shoulder. Despite the diagnostic complexity of the throwing shoulder, simple ROM measurements help to distinguish normal protective and/or performance-enhancing osseous changes from injurious soft tissue adaptations such as anterior-inferior instability and GIRD.

References

1. Lyman S, Fleisig GS, Andrews JR, Osinski ED. Effect of pitch type, pitch count, and pitching mechanics on risk of elbow and shoulder pain in youth baseball pitchers. *Am J Sports Med.* 2002;30(4):463-468.
2. Borsa PA, Laudner KG, Sauers EL. Mobility and stability adaptations in the shoulder of the overhead athlete: a theoretical and evidence-based perspective. *Sports Med.* 2008;38(1): 17-36.
3. Wilk KE, Meister K, Andrews JR. Current concepts in the rehabilitation of the overhead throwing athlete. *Am J Sports Med.* 2002;30(1):136-151.
4. Shanley E, Thigpen CA, Clark JC, et al. Changes in passive range of motion and development of glenohumeral internal rotation deficit (GIRD) in the professional pitching shoulder between spring training in two consecutive years. *J Shoulder Elbow Surg.* 2012;21(11): 1605-1612.
5. Kibler WB, Sciascia A, Thomas SJ. Glenohumeral internal rotation deficit: pathogenesis and response to acute throwing. *Sports Med Arthrosc.* 2012;20(1):34-38.

QUESTION 33

Is There a Relationship Between Shoulder and Elbow Injuries in Overhead Athletes?

Elizabeth E. Hibberd, PhD, ATC and
Joseph B. Myers, PhD, ATC

During the overhead motion used in sports such as baseball, softball, volleyball, swimming, and tennis, the forces experienced at the elbow are a result of the functioning of proximal segments, such as the shoulder and trunk. Proper functioning of the shoulder enables appropriate energy transfer in the overhead motion, allowing proximal segments to absorb the majority of the force and decreasing forces at the distal segments. Alterations in shoulder range of motion (ROM) and scapular kinematics can decrease the ability of the proximal shoulder joint to dissipate forces, leading to greater valgus stress experienced at the elbow during the overhead motion. Valgus extension overload at the elbow may cause injuries to the ulnar collateral ligament, flexor-pronator mass, medial epicondyle apophysis, ulnar nerve, posteromedial tip of the olecranon, radial head, and capitulum. Because of the influence of shoulder physical characteristics on elbow injury, it is important that clinicians assess shoulder ROM and scapular functioning when evaluating an overhead athlete with an elbow injury.

Huxel Bliven KC, ed. *Quick Questions in the Shoulder: Expert Advice in Sports Medicine* (pp 177-181).

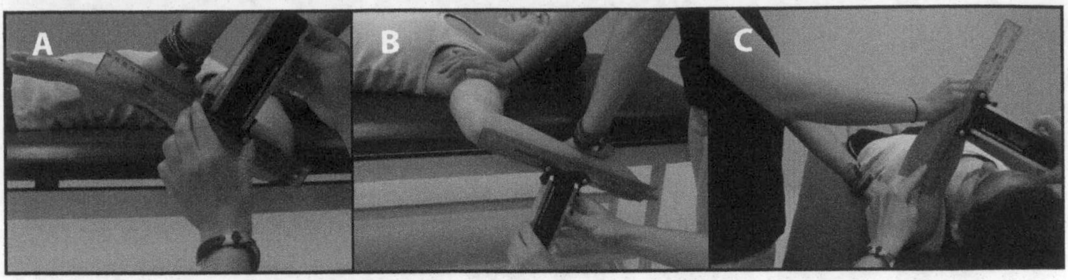

Figure 33-1. (A) Internal rotation ROM measurement. (B) External rotation ROM measurement. (C) Posterior shoulder tightness measurement.

Glenohumeral Range of Motion

A typical overhead athlete presents with greater humeral external rotation and less internal rotation on the dominant limb than on the nondominant limb. Internal rotation deficits are often offset by external rotation gain in calculating total ROM, making it necessary to measure clinical internal rotation and external rotation to note changes in one direction (Figure 33-1).

Glenohumeral internal rotation deficit (GIRD) indicates decreased internal rotation ROM on the dominant limb compared with that on the nondominant limb. GIRD has been identified as a typical physical characteristic that is displayed in overhead athletes and has been linked to the development of serious elbow injury.[1] The relationship between GIRD and elbow injury is due to biomechanical changes at the glenohumeral joint that alter the joint mechanics. Decreased internal rotation ROM leads to an anterosuperior migration of the humeral head and prevents the humeral head from remaining centered in the glenoid cavity. Subtle changes in the humeral head have significant effects on the ability of the scapular stabilizers and glenohumeral joint movers to stabilize the shoulder joint and proximally absorb forces of the overhead motion. A decreased ability of the proximal segments to absorb the forces of the overhead motion causes greater stress on the elbow. Increased forces on the elbow during repetitive overhead motions may overcome the physiological restraint abilities of the passive and/or dynamic restraints at the elbow, leading to injury, pain, and dysfunction. Recently, it was suggested that a diagnosis of pathological GIRD, which is GIRD without associated increases in external rotation ROM leading to a decrease in total ROM, is more relevant to injury risk in overhead athletes than simply evaluating GIRD.[1]

During the throwing motion, overhead athletes undergo significant external rotation ROM to generate elastic energy in the shoulder musculature to generate high rotation speeds and power during the acceleration phase. Greater external rotation ROM values have been associated with increased valgus stress at the elbow, which increases the risk of traumatic elbow injury.[2] With repetitive throwing and a high level of loading on the shoulder passive restraints, gradual stretching of the capsular collagen occurs over time, which leads to increased anterior capsular laxity. Overhead athletes may develop laxity from repetitive external rotation that manifests as anterior instability or microinstability, allowing the humeral head to translate anteriorly, preventing the humeral head from being centered within the glenoid fossa. Shoulder instability can lead to decreased functioning of the muscles of the scapular stabilizers and glenohumeral joint movers and dampen their ability to dissipate the forces at the shoulder during throwing, increasing the valgus stress at the elbow.

Overhead athletes often present with increased posterior shoulder tightness, represented by decreased horizontal adduction ROM compared with nonoverhead athletes (see Figure 33-1). The repetitive nature of the overhead motion may cause fatigue in the posterior rotator cuff muscles, which places more stress on the posterior capsule to maintain joint stability through the throwing motion. Over time, the distractive stress causes repetitive microtrauma to the posterior capsule and a fibroblastic healing response resulting in hypertrophy and contracture. A tight and hypertrophied posterior capsule can cause a shift in the arthrokinematics of the glenohumeral joint. Tightness of the posterior capsule, which also limits glenohumeral internal rotation ROM, creates an obligate anterior and superior humeral translation during shoulder flexion. Similar to alterations in external rotation ROM, the altered arthrokinematics of the shoulder joint decrease the ability of this proximal segment to absorb the forces and increase the valgus stress at the elbow during the overhead motion, which increases the risk of injury.

Although changes in ROM are typically attributed to soft tissue alterations, there are also osseous contributions to glenohumeral ROM. The bony adaptation of humeral retrotorsion results in shifting of the glenohumeral ROM, which typically presents as increased external rotation and limited internal rotation ROM, giving the deceiving appearance of having posterior shoulder hypomobility.[3] Although individuals typically exhibit some degree of asymmetry in humeral torsion, overhead athletes consistently exhibit exaggerated humeral retrotorsion in their throwing limb compared with their nondominant limb and with the dominant limbs of individuals with no history of upper extremity sport participation. This increased humeral retrotorsion in the dominant side is believed to reflect the torsion acquired from participation in throwing sports. This increased amount of retrotorsion has been linked to improved athletic performance as a result of increased elastic energy storage in the glenohumeral power-generating muscles, but it has also been identified as a risk factor for elbow injury in overhead athletes because of its influence on internal and external rotation ROM.[4] The altered kinematic chain and functioning of the shoulder increase the valgus stress at the elbow, which increases the risk of serious elbow injuries in overhead athletes.

Scapular Kinematics

The scapula is the cornerstone of upper extremity movement, and its primary role is to ensure proper position and motion for optimal shoulder function, thus decreasing forces at the elbow in overhead athletes. These alterations in scapular kinematics most likely develop in overhead athletes because of the tightness of the anterior musculature and weakness of the posterior shoulder musculature that are typical in overhead athletes. These muscle imbalances cause increased scapular protraction and decreased posterior tilting and upward rotation. Scapular positioning can also be affected by GIRD; it was previously shown that patients with GIRD of greater than 15 degrees have significantly less scapular upward rotation.[5] The observed decrease in upward rotation during active shoulder abduction is likely the result of inhibition of the dynamic scapular rotators. In addition to increasing the risk of injury at the shoulder, these alterations indicate decreased stability of the scapula, and these altered patterns of muscular coactivation lead to a decreased ability to oppose anterior humeral head migration. Together, these indicate decreased functioning of the shoulder musculature to absorb forces proximally and increased valgus stress distally at the elbow.

Conclusion

Evaluation of shoulder ROM and scapular kinematics in an athlete with elbow pain and/or injury can provide a clinician with valuable information regarding shoulder physical characteristics that may be increasing the valgus stress at the elbow. By creating stretching and strengthening interventions to address these shoulder physical characteristics, the proximal shoulder can become more effective at dissipating the forces of the overhead motion at the shoulder, thus decreasing the injury-causing valgus stress at the elbow.

References

1. Garrison JC, Cole MA, Conway JE, Macko MJ, Thigpen C, Shanley E. Shoulder range of motion deficits in baseball players with an ulnar collateral ligament tear. *Am J Sports Med.* 2012;40(11):2597-2603.
2. Fleisig GS, Andrews JR, Dillman CJ, Escamilla RF. Kinetics of baseball pitching with implications about injury mechanisms. *Am J Sports Med.* 1995;23(2):233-239.
3. Myers JB, Oyama S, Goerger BM, Rucinski TJ, Blackburn JT, Creighton RA. Influence of humeral torsion on interpretation of posterior shoulder tightness measures in overhead athletes. *Clin J Sport Med.* 2009;19(5):366-371.

4. Myers JB, Oyama S, Rucinski TJ, Creighton RA. Humeral retrotorsion in collegiate baseball pitchers with throwing-related upper extremity injury history. *Sports Health.* 2011;3(4):383-389.
5. Thomas SJ, Swanik KA, Swanik CB, Kelly JD IV. Internal rotation deficits affect scapular positioning in baseball players. *Clin Orthop Relat Res.* 2010;468(6):1551-1557.

QUESTION **34**

What Are the Optimal Shoulder Strength Ratios for Overhead Athletes, and What Strategies Should Be Implemented to Ensure Appropriate Strength Ratios?

W. Steven Tucker, PhD, ATC

Synergistic force production through a balance of agonist and antagonist muscle activation provides dynamic stabilization at the shoulder. If a joint or articulation is unable to function properly because of muscle weakness or imbalance, the kinematics of the entire shoulder complex can be compromised. As a result of the high-velocity and repetitive forces generated by overhead athletes, the shoulder complex can undergo structural and mechanical adaptations over time. These adaptations can include changes to the strength ratios of the glenohumeral joint and scapulothoracic articulation. This chapter will discuss the most common shoulder strength ratios and muscle imbalances that affect overhead athletes and examples of effective strategies to address them.

After the late cocking and acceleration phases, in which the concentrically activated internal rotators produce an extreme amount of torque at the glenohumeral joint, the eccentrically activated external rotators attempt to control the tensile

Huxel Bliven KC, ed. *Quick Questions in the Shoulder: Expert Advice in Sports Medicine* (pp 183-188).

forces to decelerate the arm. This mechanism can lead to an external/internal rotator strength ratio imbalance in which the internal rotators increase in strength while the external rotators do not. This muscle imbalance has been associated with overhead-related injuries in a variety of sports such as baseball, volleyball, tennis, and swimming. The degree of and/or an increase in the muscle imbalance may be contributing factors to injury, in that any change in the normal external/internal rotator strength ratio as a result of overhead activity may be problematic and a precursor to shoulder injury.

Determining an athlete's external/internal rotator strength ratio can be accomplished by using an isokinetic dynamometer to concentrically test the internal and external rotators through a full range of motion. It has been suggested that the external rotator strength of professional baseball pitchers should be at least 65% at 180 degrees per second and 61% at 300 degrees per second of the internal rotator strength before returning to pitching after an injury.[1] Other positions, levels of competition, and sports would likely benefit from a similar minimum external/internal strength ratio requirement. If isokinetic testing is not feasible, a hand-held dynamometer can be used with manual isometric resistance to quantify the bilateral strength of the external and internal rotators. It is recommended that overhead athletes be assessed for external/internal strength ratio, or isometric strength, in conjunction with a preparticipation examination and rehabilitation protocol, which enables the clinician to identify deficiencies or changes in the athlete's strength. An intervention plan can then be implemented to prevent future injury to the shoulder.

Normal scapular kinematics are the result of sequential scapular muscle activation patterns that stabilize and control scapular movement, enabling balanced force couples acting on the glenohumeral joint. During the overhead motion, activation of the serratus anterior, upper trapezius, middle trapezius, and lower trapezius collectively produce force couples that move the scapula into upward rotation, creating adequate room at the subacromial space. Although these muscles function together, the serratus anterior has the best mechanical advantage. During the throwing motion, activation of the serratus anterior is more than 100% of a maximum voluntary contraction (%MVC) during the late cocking and acceleration phases, while the upper trapezius is minimally activated throughout all phases.[2]

If a lack of force production from the serratus anterior occurs during overhead activity, it is compensated for by excessive activation of the upper trapezius, which causes the scapula to translate abnormally and decreases upward rotation.[3] This scapular muscle imbalance has been associated with shoulder injuries commonly associated with overhead athletes, such as instability, shoulder impingement, superior labrum anterior-to-posterior (SLAP) lesions, and rotator cuff tears. Scapular strength ratios are complicated and difficult to quantify. Static scapular upward rotation can be quantified and compared bilaterally by using a number of different instruments and techniques. Furthermore, clinicians may observe scapular dyskinesis as a result of a scapular muscle imbalance. In addition to the serratus anterior, muscle imbalances between the middle and lower trapezius can also exist with the upper trapezius.

Rehabilitation and injury-prevention protocols for overhead athletes must first address scapular muscle imbalances before rotator cuff deficiencies. Protocols should include a combination of open and closed-kinetic-chain exercises. Closed-kinetic-chain exercises elicit co-contractions of the joint-stabilizing muscles and incorporate the entire kinetic chain. Because overhead arm velocity depends on the distal-to-proximal interaction of the lower extremity, pelvis, trunk, and shoulder, upper extremity closed-kinetic-chain exercises may be particularly beneficial to overhead athletes.

For a scapular muscle imbalance, implementation should involve exercises that promote high levels of serratus anterior, middle trapezius, and lower trapezius activation and low levels of upper trapezius activation. Closed-kinetic-chain exercises tend to elicit high levels of serratus anterior activation and low levels of upper trapezius activation in healthy and injured overhead athletes. Using a Cuff Link (EFI) with the elbows flexed to perform rotational exercises in a push-up position has demonstrated the highest level of serratus anterior activation (> 68%MVC) and the lowest level of upper trapezius activation (< 10%MVC).[4] Alternatively, a BOSU ball (BOSU Fitness) can be used in place of the Cuff Link (Figure 34-1). The push-up, and variations of the push-up, elicit similar serratus anterior activation levels to the Cuff Link[4] and can be progressed from partial to full weight bearing to accommodate a patient's strength, phase of rehabilitation, and degree of difficulty.

Because of the lack of scapular stabilization, the serratus anterior can be difficult to activate at high levels with open-kinetic-chain exercises. Resistance-tubing exercises such as throwing acceleration, external rotation at 90 degrees of abduction, shoulder flexion, and scapular punch elicit high levels of serratus anterior activation.[5] However, these exercises require the shoulder to be at or above 90 degrees of elevation and should be used with caution when treating a patient with symptoms of shoulder impingement. For imbalances between the middle and lower trapezius and the upper trapezius, side-lying external rotation, side-lying forward flexion, prone horizontal abduction with external rotation, and prone extension are recommended.[6]

To address an external/internal rotator strength ratio imbalance, focus should be on activation of the posterior rotator cuff, particularly exercises that eccentrically load the external rotators. There has been limited research on exercises that activate the posterior rotator cuff because of the difficulty with which electromyography is collected. However, the previously described side-lying external rotation and prone

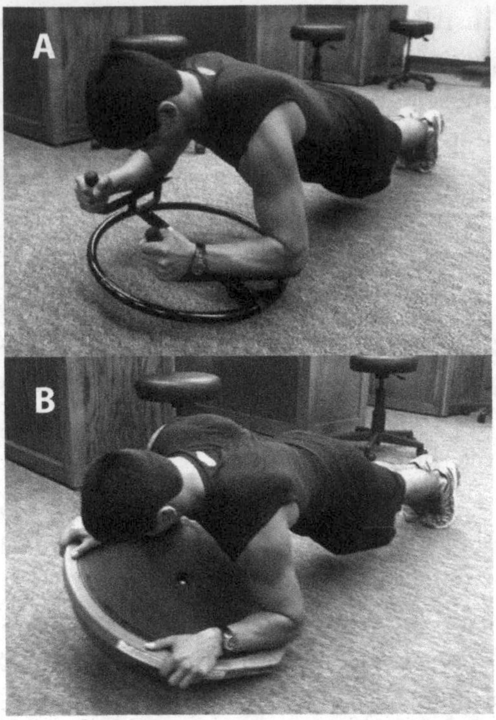

Figure 34-1. Closed-kinetic-chain exercise with the (A) Cuff Link and (B) BOSU ball. The action involves alternating the shoulders to press all edges of the apparatus down in a clockwise or counterclockwise direction.

horizontal abduction with external rotation have been found to elicit high activation levels of the posterior rotator cuff, as has the prone external rotation exercise (Figure 34-2).[7]

It is important for clinicians to accurately assess for strength ratios and muscle imbalances of the rotator cuff and scapular muscles. Although numerous muscle imbalances can exist, the most common imbalances that affect overhead athletes involve the external/internal rotator strength ratio and the serratus anterior and trapezius muscles. Once identified, exercises that address the specific deficiencies should be implemented in the rehabilitation or injury-prevention protocol. Although additional research is needed, some exercises have been found to benefit specific strength ratios and muscle imbalances in overhead athletes. Furthermore, clinicians should carefully monitor and reassess overhead athletes for changes in strength ratios and muscle imbalances.

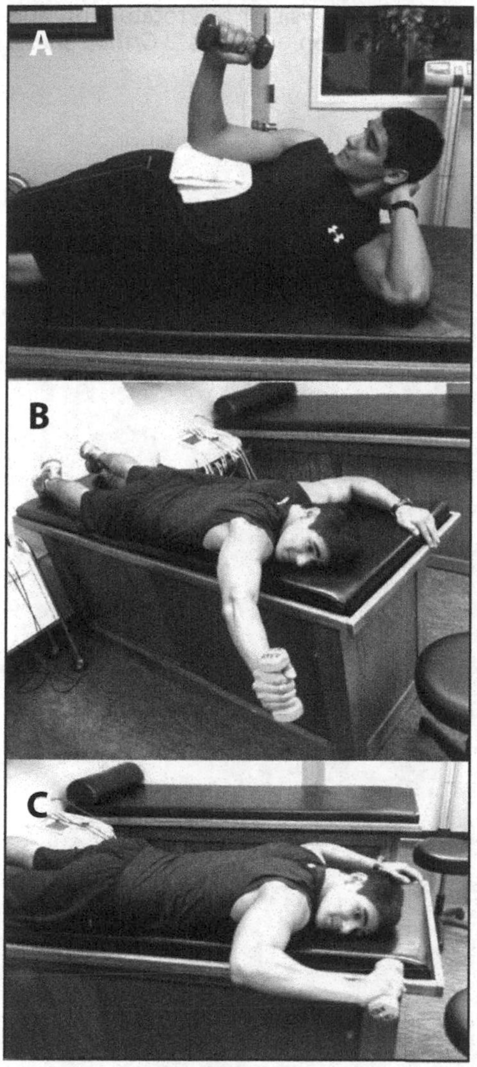

Figure 34-2. Open-kinetic-chain exercises for the posterior rotator cuff: (A) side-lying external rotation, (B) prone horizontal abduction with external rotation, and (C) prone external rotation.

References

1. Wilk KE, Andrews JR, Arrigo CA, Keirns MA, Erber DJ. The strength characteristics of internal and external rotator muscles in professional baseball pitchers. *Am J Sports Med.* 1993;21(1):61-66.
2. Gowan ID, Jobe FW, Tibone JE, Perry J, Moynes DR. A comparative electromyographic analysis of the shoulder during pitching. Professional versus amateur pitchers. *Am J Sports Med.* 1987;15(6):586-590.
3. Ludewig PM, Cook TM. Alterations in shoulder kinematics and associated muscle activity in people with symptoms of shoulder impingement. *Phys Ther.* 2000;80(3):276-291.
4. Tucker WS, Armstrong CW, Gribble PA, Timmons MK, Yeasting RA. Scapular muscle activity in overhead athletes with symptoms of secondary shoulder impingement during closed chain exercises. *Arch Phys Med Rehabil.* 2010;91(4):550-556.
5. Myers JB, Pasquale MR, Laudner KG, Sell TC, Bradley JP, Lephart SM. On-the-field resistance-tubing exercises for throwers: an electromyographic analysis. *J Athl Train.* 2005;40(1):15-22.
6. Cools AM, Dewitte V, Lanszweert F, et al. Rehabilitation of scapular muscle balance: which exercises to prescribe? *Am J Sports Med.* 2007;35(10):1744-1751.

7. Reinold MM, Wilk KE, Fleisig GS, et al. Electromyographic analysis of the rotator cuff and deltoid musculature during common shoulder external rotation exercises. *J Orthop Sports Phys Ther.* 2004;34(7):385-394.

QUESTION 35

What Are the Current Pitch Count Guidelines for Youth, Adolescent, and Adult Baseball and Softball Pitchers, and Are These Guidelines Effective in Decreasing the Number of Shoulder Injuries Experienced in These Populations?

Ellen Shanley, PhD, PT, OCS and
Amanda Arnold, PT, DPT, OCS, SCS

Pitch count guidelines were first developed in the mid-1990s as a response to growing concern for the health of young pitchers. Lyman et al[1] published a landmark study in 2002 that established a strong link between the number of pitches thrown (pitch count) and shoulder/elbow pain reported in youth baseball players. Countless studies have confirmed that excessive pitching can result in arm pain and, in some cases, lead to time-loss injuries. In 2004, the USA Baseball's Medical and Safety Advisory Committee responded by issuing safety guidelines that limited the number of pitches thrown by youth and adolescent pitchers during competition (Table 35-1).[2] Despite multiple organizations' adoption of these recommendations, upper extremity injuries in youth and adolescent baseball pitchers are on the rise.

Huxel Bliven KC, ed. *Quick Questions in the Athletic Shoulder: Expert Advice in Sports Medicine* (pp 189-193).

Table 35-1

USA Baseball Medical & Safety Advisory Committee Recommendations: Pitch Counts

Age, Years	Pitches/Game	Pitches/Week	Pitches/Season	Pitches/Year
9 to 10	50	75	1000	2000
11 to 12	75	100	1000	3000
13 to 14	75	125	1000	3000
15 to 16	90	2 games/week		
17 to 18	105	2 games/week		

Recommendations on appropriate rest days available at USA Baseball Medical & Safety Advisory website: http://web.usabaseball.com/news/article.jsp?ymd=20090813&content_id=6409508.

Adapted from USA Baseball Medical & Safety Advisory Committee. Youth baseball pitching injuries. http://web.usabaseball.com/news/article.jsp?ymd=20090813&content_id=6409508. Published November 30, 2008. Accessed December 20, 2014; and Position statement for youth baseball pitchers. American Sports Medicine Institute. http://www.asmi.org/research.php?page=research&section=positionStatement. Updated April 2013. Accessed December 20, 2014.

Shoulder injuries in baseball players are thought to be multifactorial in their development. Determining the effectiveness of pitch count recommendations in reducing overall injury rates for young baseball pitchers has been difficult. Despite clearly stated guidelines provided by USA Baseball,[2] compliance with these recommendations is inconsistent at best. One study examined coaches' knowledge of pitch count guidelines for each of the age groups they coached and found that only 43% of the questions asked were answered correctly. When polled, 73% of the coaches stated that they felt they complied with age-appropriate pitching guidelines.[3] This discrepancy in knowledge likely impacts the effectiveness of pitch count recommendations. As health care providers, we have a unique opportunity to educate and promote the importance of pitch count guidelines to the parents and coaches of the athletes we treat and to the athletes themselves. Reminding them of the perils of what can happen when an athlete throws one too many pitches may not always resonate. Emphasizing the negative effects of chronic arm fatigue on a pitcher's performance is another approach that clinicians can use to promote pitch count limits and potentially reduce shoulder injuries.

The advent of year-round baseball has also affected upper extremity injury risk, performance, and overall pitch count compliance. With multiple seasons played every year and in some cases overlapping, athletes get little time to rest and recuperate. In response to this, USA Baseball's recommendations include weekly, seasonal, and yearly pitch counts that were designed to account for the aggregate stresses placed on a pitcher's arm over the course of 1 year. These pitch count recommendations have been widely disseminated and accepted as beneficial for the athletes, but they are poorly enforced.[2] A pitcher can stay within his or her pitch count limits on the Little League team and then go pitch for a travel team the next day without repercussions. Each pitch thrown places additional stresses across an athlete's arm that require adequate time and rest to recover. One means of preventing this lapse in communication is through regular medical screening. Athletic trainers and medical support staff should have access to both medical and playing histories on each of the players they work with. The number of teams for which youth athletes play and the number of positions they play often vary more than those of their skeletally mature counterparts. Frequent growth spurts also contribute to overuse because they can inherently weaken bony and muscular structures in young athletes. Without proper rest and variation in movement, fatigue will set in, thereby increasing that player's risk for shoulder injuries.[4]

Baseball and softball pitchers demonstrate similar risk for developing throwing-related shoulder injuries attributable to overuse.[5] Despite this fact, pitch count guidelines in fast-pitch softball are in their infancy, likely because of common misconceptions concerning the relative safety of fast-pitch softball. Youth softball pitchers often throw in excess of 1200 to 1500 pitches over the course of 3 days with little time to rest or recuperate. This pitch count is 10 to 20 times higher than that recommended for baseball pitchers of the same age.[5]

Few research studies have sought to examine the biomechanics behind the windmill or under-handed pitching motion and the effects thereof. Current literature suggests that windmill pitchers sustain large forces across their shoulder and elbow joints while pitching, approximately 70% to 95% of the forces experienced in baseball pitching motions. To balance these forces and prevent injury, fast-pitch pitchers require as much if not more strength in their arm muscles than their baseball counterparts.[5] Health care practitioners, including strength and conditioning coaches, should be aware of the unique stresses placed on the arms of fast-pitch pitchers and should adjust their treatment plans accordingly. Emphasizing scapular control and rotator cuff strength can assist in counteracting the large distraction forces experienced at the shoulder during a windmill pitch.

A variety of governing bodies exist for the sport of fast-pitch softball, the most common of which are the Amateur Softball Association and the United States Specialty Sports Association (USSSA). Unfortunately, neither of these groups (or any of their counterparts) has officially endorsed or disseminated softball-specific pitch count guidelines. The USSSA suggested maximums on the number of games that a youth pitcher (7 to 14 years) should pitch, but actual pitch counts were not included. The fast-pitch softball pitch count guidelines listed in this chapter

Table 35-2 **Fast-Pitch Softball Recommendations: Pitch Counts**		
Age, Years	**Pitches/Game**	**Pitches/Weekend**
8 to 10	50	80
10 to 12	65	95
13 to 14	80	195
15+	100	240

Adapted from Softball Injury Prevention. University of Florida Orthopaedics and Rehabilitation. http://www.ortho.ufl.edu/sites/ortho.ufl.edu/files/handouts/Softball-Injury-Prevention.pdf.

(Table 35-2) were compiled from the scientific literature available to date in an effort to decrease the number of arm injuries experienced by young softballers.[5]

As with any skilled movement, young athletes require copious amounts of repetition to effectively master the windmill pitching motion. Unlike overhead throwing in baseball, not every fast-pitch softball player can replicate the required pitching motion at the same rate. Many invested parties argue against pitch count guidelines in fast-pitch softball. They believe that it will alter the way the game is played. The current research states that up to 85% of injuries sustained by softball pitchers are related to overuse.[4] Pitch count guidelines are one way to limit exposure and potentially affect the overall health of these athletes. Fast-pitch pitchers will inherently throw more pitches per game, season, and year than their baseball equivalents, even if the prescribed pitch count guidelines are enforced. This fact implies that endurance, while important in baseball, is imperative in fast-pitch softball. Health care professionals can affect injury risk in this population by emphasizing both strength and endurance in the training programs they design. Velocity, accuracy, and situational decision making are all affected when an athlete is fatigued. Improved global and muscular endurance has the potential to positively influence shoulder injury risk and improve overall performance factors.

Some believe that throwing and pitching at a young age is a necessary part of development for an athlete, but how much is too much? When does the risk outweigh the benefits? Pitch count recommendations aim to encourage participation while minimizing an athlete's risk for an arm injury that could plague him or her throughout his or her career, in some cases prematurely ending it. For these guidelines to effectively decrease the number and severity of shoulder injuries sustained in these populations, coaches, parents, and the athletes themselves must increase their knowledge concerning the effects of excessive throwing without sufficient recovery. Variation in sport, sufficient rest, and careful monitoring of any arm pain or soreness is imperative if baseball and softball injury rates are to decrease in the next 10 years.

References

1. Lyman S, Fleisig GS, Andrews JR, Osinski ED. Effect of pitch type, pitch count, and pitching mechanics on risk of elbow and shoulder pain in youth baseball pitchers. *Am J Sports Med.* 2002;30(4):463-468.
2. USA Baseball Medical & Safety Advisory Committee. Youth baseball pitching injuries. http://web.usabaseball.com/news/article.jsp?ymd=20090813&content_id=6409508. Published November 30, 2008. Accessed December 20, 2014.
3. Fazarale JJ, Magnussen RA, Pedroza AD, Kaeding CC, Best TM, Classie J. Knowledge of and compliance with pitch count recommendations: a survey of youth baseball coaches. *Sports Health*. 2012;4(3):202-204.
4. Hill JL, Humphries B, Weidner T, Newton RU. Female collegiate windmill pitchers: influences to injury incidence. *J Strength Cond Res.* 2004;18(3):426-431.
5. Krajnik S, Fogarty KJ, Yard EE, Comstock RD. Shoulder injuries in US high school baseball and softball athletes, 2005-2008. *Pediatrics.* 2010;125(3):497-501.

QUESTION **36**

What Are Important Considerations in Managing the Adolescent Baseball Pitcher With Shoulder Pain?

Sue Falsone, PT, MS, SCS, ATC, CSCS, COMT;
Gail P. Parr, PhD, ATC; and Kellie C. Huxel Bliven, PhD, ATC

Identifying risk factors is an important component in preventing the onset or reducing the severity of injuries sustained by athletes. Injuries attributed to throwing overhead are relatively common for athletes of all ages. However, the risk factors for such injuries can vary according to age. The risk factors for the adolescent baseball pitcher are notably different from those of the adult pitcher. This chapter presents information pertaining to risk factors and injuries to the adolescent baseball pitcher. The intent is for management of the adolescent pitcher to begin with this knowledge base in an effort to decrease the onset and severity of injury.

The number of pitches thrown in a game, the number of pitches thrown in the season, and the rest period between throwing sessions are modifiable risk factors that can affect the adolescent pitcher. Policies have been established in Little League baseball regarding these factors. Although these policies are beneficial, they are not sufficient to reduce injuries sustained by adolescent pitchers. To reduce

Huxel Bliven KC, ed. *Quick Questions in the Shoulder: Expert Advice in Sports Medicine* (pp 195-197).

a young athlete's susceptibility to injury, the clinician must have an understanding of shoulder anatomy of the adolescent and the biomechanics of throwing, including the role of the dynamic and static stabilizers in areas other than the shoulder (ie, the elbow, the trunk and spine, and the lower extremities).

The physical immaturity of the shoulder complex is largely responsible for the incidence of injury to the adolescent pitcher. One unique feature of the adolescent shoulder is that the epiphyseal plates remain open much longer than we may realize. The average age for closure of the proximal humerus is 17 to 18 years, that of the glenoid is 16 to 18 years, and that of the clavicle is 18 to 20 years.[1,2] Another attribute that can have negative consequences for the adolescent pitcher is that the proximal epiphyseal plate is weaker than the surrounding ligaments. A third characteristic of the adolescent shoulder is the underdeveloped musculature in the region. These 3 features are nonmodifiable risk factors for the adolescent pitcher.[1] The combination of these factors with the significant rotational and shearing forces associated with the overhead throwing mechanism can result in injuries unique to the adolescent pitcher. An explanation of the forces generated during the 6 phases of throwing is beyond the scope of this chapter. However, the clinician would be well served to understand the mechanics and forces sustained throughout the various phases of the overhead throw.

In addition to being able to identify modifiable and nonmodifiable risk factors, the clinician must be familiar with warning signs that suggest potential injury. The proximal humeral epiphysis is a common site of injury in adolescent pitchers. The torsional loads associated with maximum external rotation in the cocking phase of throwing can widen the proximal humeral physis. Proximal humeral epiphysiolysis, or Little League shoulder, is an overuse injury that primarily affects 11- to 14-year-olds. It is characterized by a gradual onset of upper arm pain and decreased performance. The hallmark sign of this injury is point tenderness on the lateral aspect of the proximal humerus.[1,2]

The lack of muscular development in the shoulder complex can predispose the adolescent pitcher to rotator cuff dysfunction and atraumatic glenohumeral instability. Rotator cuff injuries in adolescents differ from those seen in the adult pitcher. In adults, the primary mechanism is impingement, whereas in adolescents, dysfunction of the rotator cuff is attributed to undersurface tears from overuse and the forces associated with throwing.[2] Characteristic of this condition is pain at ball release and throughout deceleration and follow-through. Tears of the rotator cuff are much less common in adolescents than adult pitchers; even still, they should be recognized as a possible injury.

In a similar manner, superior labral anterior-to-posterior (SLAP) lesions are more common in adults than in adolescents, but the absence of muscular development in adolescents can compromise dynamic stabilization of the shoulder.[2] Signs and symptoms of a SLAP injury include deep shoulder pain during the cocking phase of throwing, decreased throwing velocity, and popping or catching during rotational movements.

In general, the clinician should initiate management as soon as the adolescent pitcher presents with any signs or symptoms at the shoulder and any dysfunction along the entire kinetic chain. Signs and symptoms specific to the shoulder include gradual onset of upper arm pain that increases with throwing, decreased performance (eg, velocity and accuracy), altered glenohumeral range of motion and laxity, weak and painful external rotation, and poor rotator cuff and scapular muscle activation and control.[1]

Physical measures along the entire kinetic chain should be examined to identify dysfunctions contributing to and causing the pain. Shoulder-related issues include alterations in glenohumeral range of motion, posterior shoulder tightness, rotator cuff and scapular muscle imbalance and weakness, and scapular dyskinesis. Trunk, spine, and lower extremity–related issues include decreased trunk, hip, and ankle range of motion, decreased quantity and quality of spinal mobility, and atypical spinal curves. Each of these factors can provide insight pertaining to the use of the trunk, spine, and lower extremities during complex throwing movement patterns. For example, limits in range of motion, inadequate strength, and strength imbalances in these areas can have significant implications for executing the proper mechanics in the upper component of the kinetic chain, including the shoulder complex and upper extremities.

The clinician is faced with a variety of challenges, including understanding the mechanics of the throwing motion, recognizing impairments or dysfunctions along the entire kinetic chain, and being familiar with signs and symptoms of potential shoulder injuries. Perhaps the biggest challenge is recognizing that the adolescent is experiencing rapid changes in growth and development. As such, the management of an adolescent pitcher is an ongoing process that must be assessed and re-evaluated on a continual and constant basis to provide the best possible care for the individual.

References

1. Shanley E, Thigpen C. Throwing injuries in the adolescent athlete. *Int J Sports Phys Ther.* 2013;8(5):630-640.
2. Zaremski JL, Krabak BJ. Shoulder injuries in the skeletally immature baseball pitcher and recommendations for the prevention of injury. *PM R.* 2012;4(7):509-516.

QUESTION 37

What Are the Components of a Safe and Effective Return-to-Throwing Progression for Pitchers?

Sue Falsone, PT, MS, SCS, ATC, CSCS, COMT

Returning a pitcher to full participation after injury requires implementing an individualized throwing-progression program of distinct phases. The implementation of such a program requires the clinician to understand how forces are imparted on tissues as well as the healing process mechanisms and timetable. This knowledge is essential to ensure minimal setbacks and reduce the likelihood of reinjury. This chapter outlines considerations for the clinician in implementing the interval throwing program for a pitcher.

When a pitcher is able to demonstrate full range of motion, dynamic stabilization, muscular strength, and endurance, the clinician should consult the physician regarding initiation of an interval throwing program. An interval throwing program is intended to have the pitcher progress through phases of return to throwing, return to pitching, increased intensity of pitching, and simulated game play.[1] In each phase, it is important to integrate sport-specific and whole-body activities to restore functional movement, particularly at the injury site; to continue performing warm-up and maintenance exercises; and to ensure proper throwing mechanics.[2]

Huxel Bliven KC, ed. *Quick Questions in the Shoulder: Expert Advice in Sports Medicine* (pp 199-202).

During the course of the program, reducing the risk of recurrence of symptoms is essential. Individualization of a program is key to progressing with minimal, if any, setbacks. As a rule, any recurrence of symptoms, particularly inflammation in the injured joint or muscle and continued soreness after throwing, indicates that the athlete is progressing too fast and must return to an earlier phase in the program.

Many of the recommendations for implementing interval throwing programs are based on experience and theory, with minimal research support. Regardless, several important variables must be considered to implement a safe and effective return-to-throwing program. These variables include throwing distance, number of throws, throwing intensity, frequency of throwing, throwing from flat ground to mound, types of pitches thrown, and position of the throwing partner.

Although there is debate about throwing distance, it is somewhat established that pitchers should begin by throwing short distances (45 feet) and increase distances to 180 feet by 15-foot increments over a period of 4 to 6 weeks on flat ground. The controversy about throwing distance revolves around the "long toss" or maximum distance of throws (> 120 feet). In a study comparing pitching and long-toss mechanics, it was found that hard, horizontal, flat-ground throws were biomechanically similar to pitching; however, maximum-distance throws detrimentally altered pitching mechanics.[3] This finding suggests that caution should be used with maximum-distance throws.[3] It is important to recognize a relationship between throwing distance and velocity (miles per hour) up to a point (undefined), after which distance (typically > 150 feet) is achieved at the cost of proper pitching mechanics. The consequence is increased force and torque through the shoulder and elbow. Published protocols that describe appropriate distances should be used as a guide when determining maximum throwing distance. It should also be noted that the minimum and maximum throwing distances should be shorter for youth pitchers.[1]

Although most published interval throwing programs are based on the number of throws in each step of the progression, recent trends have shifted the focus to time spent throwing instead of number of throws for each step of the interval throwing program. Regardless of the approach, the clinician must monitor and appropriately adjust throwing intensity, volume, and frequency. Knowledge of the pitcher's preinjury maximal throwing velocity can be used to calculate percent effort and throwing velocity throughout the program by using a radar gun. Most programs begin with short tosses at no more than 50% effort. When an appropriate base is established, intensity should progress from 70% to 80% and then to 90% effort, throwing fastballs on flat ground. The clinician must realize that the ability of the pitcher to estimate throwing effort is poor. In one study, pitchers were instructed to throw at 50% effort; radar gun measurements indicated that throws were an average of 83% of the pitcher's maximum speed.[4]

After the establishment of an appropriate throwing base, throwing volume and frequency should become the focus of the program. In this phase, consideration must be given to the pitcher's preinjury throwing profile. For example, the type of pitcher (eg, starting or relief) influences the number of throws completed on a routine basis and the level that must be attained to return to competition. While starters and relievers may throw every day or throw 2 days and rest 1 day, starters may throw with more varied intensity, distance, and volume than relievers. As such, the time required to develop an acceptable endurance level can vary depending on the type of pitcher and the different types of pitches thrown (eg, fastball, breaking ball, curve, change-up).

During the interval throwing program, the fastball should be used initially. Other types of pitches should not be introduced until later in the program. Research suggests that the order of types of pitches performed should progress from fastballs to change-ups and then to curve and breaking balls. This order is based on the loads and torque applied to the shoulder and elbow.[5] Throwing only fastballs for an extended period of time protects the arm and reduces the additional stress of breaking balls while the pitcher builds up arm strength to safely return to the mound. When a pitcher has worked up to the maximum distance with a fastball throw, the next step is to work back down to 60 feet (approximately the distance from the mound). When the pitcher is able to throw 80% to 90% of his or her velocity at 60 feet on flat ground without a recurrence of symptoms, the next step is throwing down before progressing to breaking balls. Throwing down involves the throwing partner going from a standing position to a crouched position, similar to that of a catcher. The progression to a downward-slope throw helps prepare for the mound-throwing phase. The pitcher should include breaking balls from flat ground before attempting them from the mound.

When a pitcher has completed the flat-ground phase without pain, pitching from the mound can be initiated. Mound sessions should follow the schedule for what the athlete would normally do (starters vs relievers). The pitcher should throw only fastballs for the first several outings. It is important to establish confidence and control with the fastball before introducing other pitches.

Game-day intensity is difficult, if not impossible, to replicate. Simulated games, in which the pitcher throws to live hitters and the pitch count is monitored, are the closest to pitching in an actual game. In a simulated game, rest should be scheduled after several hitters to mimic pitching an inning.

The next phase of the progression, often referred to as a "rehab game," is pitching in an actual game but at a lower level (eg, AAA or AA in professional baseball). The necessary number and frequency of rehab games is determined primarily by the type of pitcher (eg, reliever or starter) and the length of time out of competition.

After successful completion of this phase, return to game competition is the final step.

Conclusion

Return-to-throwing programs should be individualized, and progression should be based on a variety of factors. Manipulating one variable at a time during the return-to-throwing process can significantly help the clinician implement a successful, progressive throwing program. In addition, it is important to maintain consistent communication with the athlete, physician, and pitching coach to facilitate a smooth progression through the program.

References

1. Axe M, Hurd W, Snyder-Mackler L. Data-based interval throwing programs for baseball players. *Sports Health*. 2009;1(2):145-153.
2. Reinold MM, Wilk KE, Reed J, Crenshaw K, Andrews JR. Interval sport programs: guidelines for baseball, tennis, and golf. *J Orthop Sports Phys Ther*. 2002;32(6):293-298.
3. Fleisig GS, Bolt B, Fortenbaugh D, Wilk KE, Andrews JR. Biomechanical comparison of baseball pitching and long-toss: implications for training and rehabilitation. *J Orthop Sports Phys Ther*. 2011;41(5):296-303.
4. Slenker NR, Limpisvasti O, Mohr K, Aguinaldo A, Elattrache NS. Biomechanical comparison of the interval throwing program and baseball pitching: upper extremity loads in training and rehabilitation. *Am J Sports Med*. 2014;42(5):1226-1232.
5. Fleisig GS, Kingsley DS, Loftice JW, et al. Kinetic comparison among the fastball, curveball, change-up, and slider in collegiate baseball pitchers. *Am J Sports Med*. 2006;34(3):423-430.

QUESTION 38

What Are Important Considerations in Managing Chronic Glenohumeral Microinstability in the Tennis Athlete?

Josie L. Harding, BS, ATC, AT;
Marilyn (Hintz) Kaminski, MS, ATC/L, CSCS; and
Barton E. Anderson, MS, AT, ATC

Tennis has seen a recent growth in popularity over the past 2 decades, with tens of millions of players throughout the world.[1] With increased participation, improved racquet technology, and unique sport demands, tennis players are at risk for musculoskeletal overuse injuries. The tennis serve requires a large amount of glenohumeral (GH) joint motion, placing significant demands on the joint's static and dynamic structures to maintain stability. Upper extremity overuse injuries account for 20% to 49% of injuries in tennis players.[1]

A variety of factors, including altered range of motion, poor dynamic stability, and abnormal muscle activation patterns, can lead to chronic microinstability and shoulder pathology. It is essential to address factors that contribute to GH microinstability through a comprehensive rehabilitation program. For tennis

Huxel Bliven KC, ed. *Quick Questions in the Shoulder: Expert Advice in Sports Medicine* (pp 203-208).

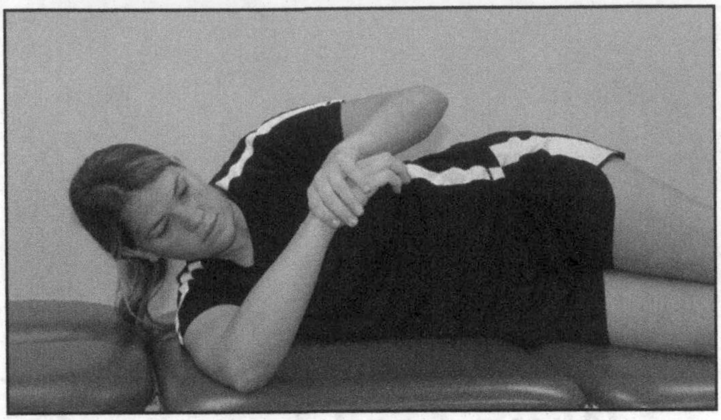

Figure 38-1. Sleeper stretch.

athletes with GH microinstability, an effective treatment approach must achieve the following goals:

- Restore normal GH rotation and arthrokinematics, especially internal rotation
- Improve GH and scapular dynamic stabilization
- Restore sequenced muscle activation patterns of the core and upper extremity

Range of Motion

The cocking phase of the tennis serve requires extreme amounts of GH external rotation, similar to that in other overhead sports.[2] In addition, significant eccentric contraction of the posterior rotator cuff muscles occurs during the deceleration phase of the serve. These ranges and forces lead to adaptive changes that result in increased GH external rotation and decreased internal rotation compared with the nondominant shoulder.[2] Such changes create an altered axis of rotation at the GH joint, disrupting the normal length-tension relationships of the rotator cuff and scapular stabilizers.[3] Therefore, restoration of normal GH rotation is imperative for any shoulder rehabilitation program.

Range of motion assessment should include a comparison of the total arc of motion available bilaterally; clinicians should be concerned with differences of greater than 10 degrees.[2] If significant restrictions are found, a variety of techniques to improve GH internal rotation can be used, including posterior humeral glides to help re-establish normal arthrokinematics and self-directed posterior capsule stretching (Figure 38-1).[3]

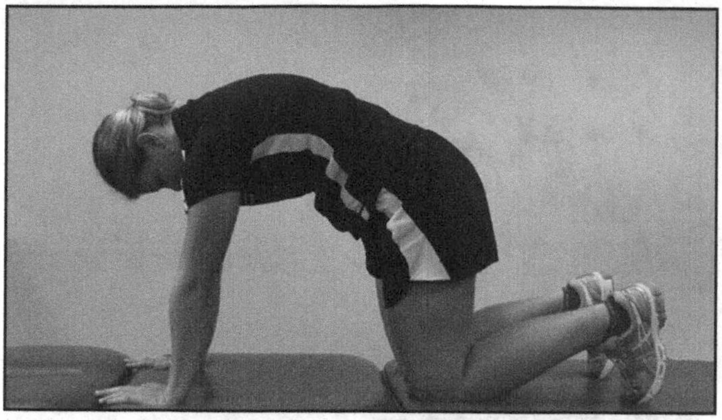

Figure 38-2. Quadruped protraction.

Dynamic Stabilization

In tennis athletes, appropriate dynamic stabilization can often be lost, resulting in poor force-couple activation at both the scapulothoracic and GH joints and the development of GH microinstability. Exercises to restore normal scapular and GH stability must be integrated before functional or sport-specific exercises are implemented.[4]

Muscular force couples maintain dynamic control of the shoulder complex. The levator scapulae, trapezius, rhomboids, and serratus anterior muscles couple together to control the movements and stability of the scapulothoracic joint. Scapular stabilization, in turn, helps to maintain rotator cuff length-tension relationships, resulting in improved force production and improved GH stability.[5]

Exercises to improve dynamic stability of the shoulder should begin with closed-chain activities to help improve coactivation of scapular stabilizers and rotator cuff muscles.[3] For example, quadruped protraction can be used to begin the activation of scapular and GH stabilizers in the closed kinetic chain. Focus should be placed on co-contraction of the rotator cuff musculature along with the middle and lower trapezius, serratus anterior, and rhomboids. Progression from the quadruped to the plank position will increase the stability demand on the shoulder, and unstable surfaces such as foam pads or wobble boards can also be used to increase dynamic stability (Figures 38-2 to 38-4).

Once stability of the scapula and GH joint is re-established in the closed kinetic chain, open-kinetic-chain activities can be implemented to restore dynamic stability with GH movement. Example exercises include active shoulder motions of flexion, external rotation, and abduction; scapular retractions; and traditional elastic tubing activities.[3] A wide variety of therapeutic exercises can be used to improve scapular and GH joint stability.

Figure 38-3. Plank.

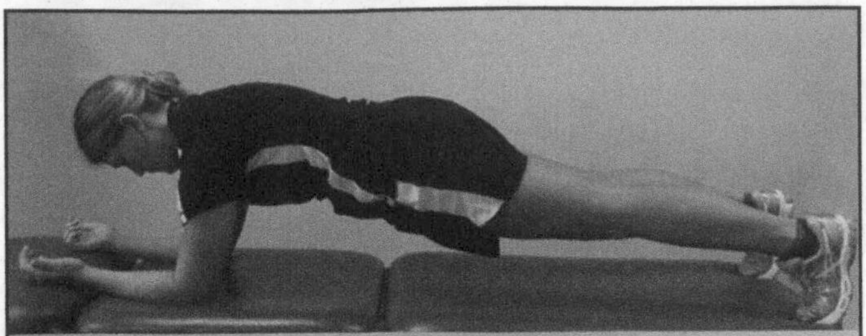

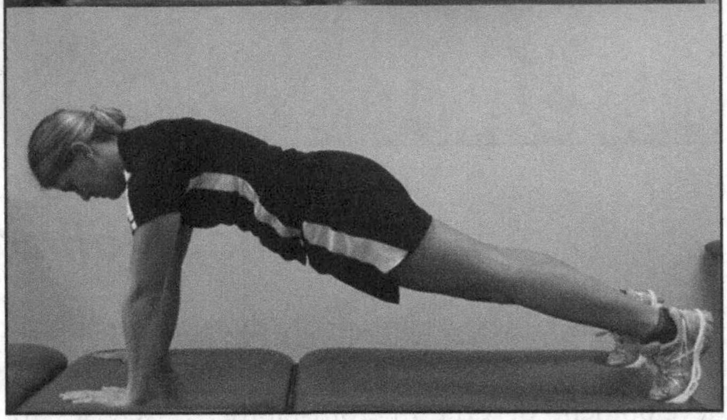

Figure 38-4. Unstable plank.

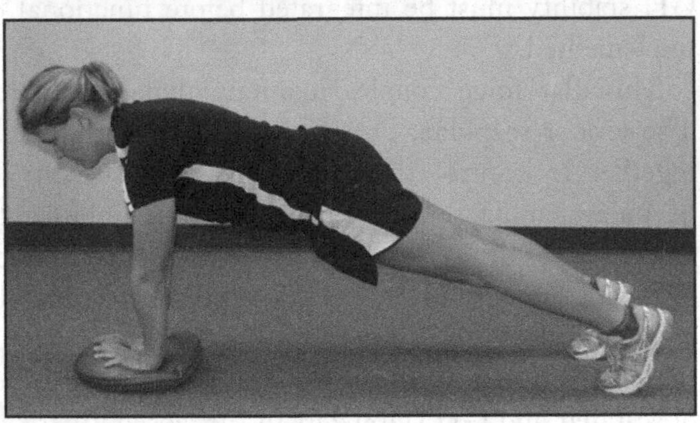

Muscle Activation Patterns

Once normal range of motion and dynamic GH and scapular stability have been restored, attention can be turned to the integration of sequenced muscle activation patterns to promote optimal transfer of energy along the kinetic chain.[5] Of primary importance is the integration of core muscle activation to produce the proximal stability necessary for sport-specific shoulder movements.[5]

The core serves 2 primary functions: providing lumbopelvic stability and serving as the foundation for the transfer of forces. The co-contraction of the transverse abdominis and multifidus increases intra-abdominal pressure and tension within the thoracolumbar fascia, increasing lumbar spine stabilization.[5] Activation of the rectus abdominis and abdominal oblique muscles also provides postural support

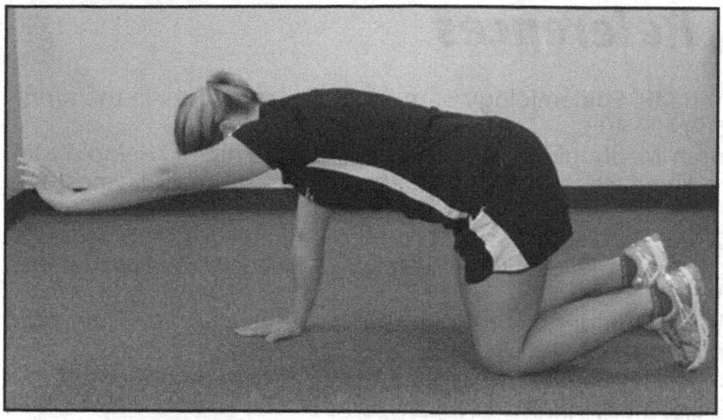

Figure 38-5. Quadruped extension.

and stabilization during limb movement. Just as GH function depends on good scapular stability, shoulder function and power depend on adequate core stability. Exercises such as quadruped shoulder extensions can be used to begin to restore appropriate muscle activation patterns. During the quadruped extension, the focus should be placed on establishing good spinal alignment and stability, followed by shoulder flexion; spinal alignment and scapular stability must be maintained throughout the movement (Figure 38-5). This deliberate sequence helps to establish a motor pattern of proximal stability for distal movements.[5]

Quadruped extensions can be progressed to higher-level activities, including chops/lifts, diagonal/rotational patterned movements, and plyometric exercise.[3]

Sport-Specific Activities and Return to Play

Once the initial goals of normalized range of motion, improved dynamic stability, and restored muscle activation patterns are achieved, a progression back to sport can be initiated. A return to play for tennis should begin with the athlete simulating strokes without ball contact followed by forehand and backhand strokes with a lightweight ball (ie, foam or whiffle ball) and then progressing to strokes with a standard tennis ball.[2] The velocity and distance of the strokes should be progressed within each phase, and emphasis should be placed on proper stroke mechanics.

Tennis athletes represent a growing population at risk for musculoskeletal overuse injuries. The unique sport demands and extreme ranges of motion often result in altered range of motion, poor dynamic stability, and altered muscle activation patterns, resulting in GH microinstability and pain. Effective treatment approaches for tennis players with chronic microinstability should focus on eliminating range of motion deficits, improving dynamic stability, and restoring normal muscle activation patterns.

References

1. Abrams GD, Renstrom PA, Safran MR. Epidemiology of musculoskeletal injury in the tennis player. *Br J Sports Med.* 2012;46(7):492-498.
2. Ellenbecker TS, Roetert EP, Safran M. Shoulder injuries in tennis. In: Wilk KE, Reinold MM, Andrews JR, eds. *The Athlete's Shoulder.* 2nd ed. Philadelphia, PA: Churchill Livingstone; 2009:429-444.
3. Hoffman S, Hughes C, Riddle G, Ross O. Neuromuscular control exercises for shoulder instability. In: Wilk KE, Reinold MM, Andrews JR, eds. *The Athlete's Shoulder.* 2nd ed. Philadelphia, PA: Churchill Livingstone; 2009:627-638.
4. van der Hoeven H, Kibler WB. Shoulder injuries in tennis players. *Br J Sports Med.* 2006;40(5):435-440; discussion 440.
5. Kibler WB, Sciascia A, Thomas SJ. Glenohumeral internal rotation deficit: pathogenesis and response to acute throwing. *Sports Med Arthrosc.* 2012;20(1):34-38.

QUESTION 39

Which Training Modifications Can Be Advantageous in Reducing Shoulder Pain and Preventing Shoulder Injury in the Competitive Swimmer?

Angela Tate, PT, PhD, Cert. MDT

Because of the repetitive nature of their training, swimmers may perform 4000 shoulder revolutions when swimming 10,000 meters/day, and hence they incur a high incidence of shoulder pain. Studies have found that 40% to 91% of competitive swimmers in the youth through masters age groups incur pain.[1,2] Risk factors associated with shoulder pain have been identified,[2] and evidence-based prevention/intervention considerations fall into 3 broad categories: in-water training, swimming technique, and dry land training.

With respect to in-water training, the greatest risk factor for shoulder pain is high training volume, which has been shown to produce supraspinatus tendinopathy.[1] Although guidelines for optimal training yardage are not available, Sein et al[1] performed magnetic resonance imaging studies on the shoulders of elite swimmers aged 13 to 25 years and found that those who swam more than 35 km or 15 hours per week were more likely to have tendinopathy than those swimming fewer yards and hours, and all swimmers who trained more than 20 hours had tendinopathy. Based on this finding, recommendations for yardage reduction may be appropriate

Huxel Bliven KC, ed. *Quick Questions in the Shoulder: Expert Advice in Sports Medicine* (pp 209-212).

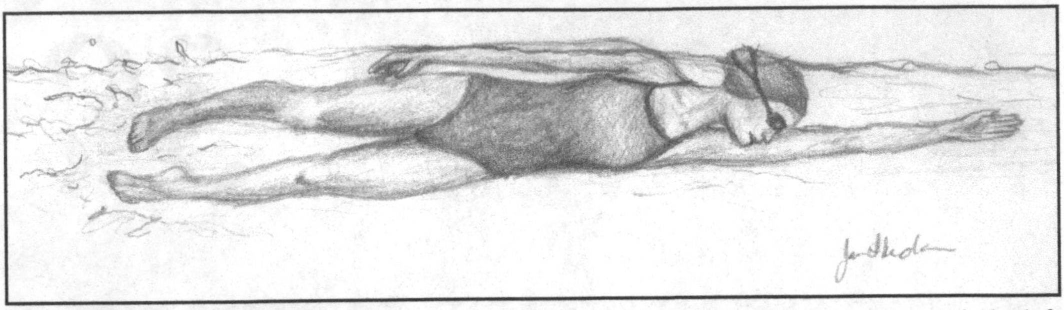

Figure 39-1. Swimmer performing a kicking sequence in the left side-lying position with the left arm overhead as part of a kick/pull drill. (Illustration by Jan Ikeda. Reprinted with permission.)

for the swimmer with painful shoulders. By assisting with propulsion, the use of fins is also advocated to reduce the load on the shoulders. In addition, the use of kickboards should be limited because sustained overhead positioning may provoke pain or increase pain in already symptomatic individuals, as may the use of tethered devices such as parachutes and additional clothing to promote drag. Kick/pull drills prevent sustained bilateral overhead activity and may be preferable to the use of kickboards. Kick/pull drills involve the swimmer completing a specified number of kicks in the side-lying position with one arm abducted overhead, followed by a brief pull sequence, and then repeating the kicking on the contralateral side (Figure 39-1).

An assessment of swimming techniques, which involves individual stroke analysis, is beyond the scope of this chapter but should be an ongoing process by a qualified coach or in conjunction with a clinician who has competitive swimming experience. The treating clinician is encouraged to obtain video clips taken during practice or competition to assess for faulty stroke mechanics. If errors are present, clinicians should take the time to explain or demonstrate to the athlete the anatomy of the shoulder and how an arm entry with shoulder internal rotation or arm crossing midline, for example, can contribute to subacromial impingement and shoulder pain.

If a swimmer is incurring shoulder pain, the initial assessment should include questioning about the current training regime, including number of practices per day and per week, yardage, and time spent performing both dry land and in-water activities. A detailed description of dry land training should be obtained, including cross training, specific stretches performed as well as parameters for stretching (repetitions and time held), and strengthening exercises. Particular attention should be aimed at determining whether repetitive resisted activities, such as bench presses, overhead presses, and push-ups, are being performed at or above shoulder level. Because swimmers already perform thousands of repetitions of shoulder elevation during practice, which is a risk factor for shoulder impingement, additional

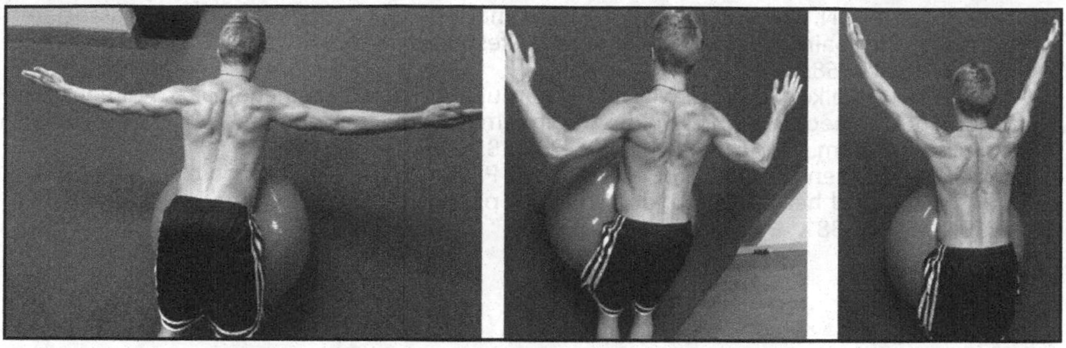

Figure 39-2. T, W, and Y exercises performed prone on a physioball to strengthen scapular muscles.

resisted elevation is not advised in the presence of pain. In addition, if the rotator cuff, which functions to center the humeral head in the glenoid, is weak or inhibited as a result of pain, elevation exercises may allow superior translation of the humeral head by the deltoid, which may further contribute to shoulder impingement.[3] A program to first strengthen the rotator cuff in a neutral position should be incorporated, as should pain-free scapular stabilization training with an emphasis on the middle and lower trapezius because they are frequently found to be weak.

Because swimmers' shoulders are typically hypermobile, stretching exercises should be limited to areas of tightness typically found in swimmers; specifically, they should address the forward head and rounded shoulders posture. Lynch et al[4] found favorable changes in swimmers' posture with the use of self pectoralis stretching and chin tucks, both performed on a foam roll in conjunction with serratus anterior and middle and lower trapezius strengthening. Forearm push-up plus exercises were used, as were prone T, W, and Y exercises on a physioball (Figure 39-2).[4]

Cross-training and core endurance activities involving limited upper extremity use should also be considered as methods for improving cardiovascular endurance and providing improved force transmission through the kinetic chain. Although prospective studies have not been performed to determine the effect of cross training, swimmers participating in walking, running, and soccer were found to have less shoulder pain than their counterparts not engaged in cross-training activities.[2] More research is needed to determine safe levels of exposure with respect to in water training and the optimization of training methods to reduce the occurrence of shoulder pain and injury.

References

1. Sein ML, Walton J, Linklater J, et al. Shoulder pain in elite swimmers: primarily due to swim-volume-induced supraspinatus tendinopathy. *Br J Sports Med.* 2010;44(2):105-113.

2. Tate A, Turner GN, Knab SE, Jorgensen C, Strittmatter A, Michener LA. Risk factors associated with shoulder pain and disability across the lifespan of competitive swimmers. *J Athl Train.* 2012;47(2):149-158.
3. McClure PW, Bialker J, Neff N, Williams G, Karduna A. Shoulder function and 3-dimensional kinematics in people with shoulder impingement syndrome before and after a 6-week exercise program. *Phys Ther.* 2004;84(9):832-848.
4. Lynch SS, Thigpen CA, Mihalik JP, Prentice WE, Padua D. The effects of an exercise intervention on forward head and rounded shoulder postures in elite swimmers. *Br J Sports Med.* 2010;44(5):376-381.

FINANCIAL DISCLOSURES

Barton E. Anderson has no financial or proprietary interest in the materials presented herein.

Dr. Amanda Arnold has no financial or proprietary interest in the materials presented herein.

Sue Falsone has no financial or proprietary interest in the materials presented herein.

Bryce W. Gaunt has no financial or proprietary interest in the materials presented herein.

Josie L. Harding has no financial or proprietary interest in the materials presented herein.

Dr. Elizabeth E. Hibberd has no financial or proprietary interest in the materials presented herein.

Dr. Kellie C. Huxel Bliven has no financial or proprietary interest in the materials presented herein.

Marilyn (Hintz) Kaminski has no financial or proprietary interest in the materials presented herein.

Dr. Martin J. Kelley has no financial or proprietary interest in the materials presented herein.

Joseph H. Kostuch has no financial or proprietary interest in the materials presented herein.

Dr. Kevin Laudner has no financial or proprietary interest in the materials presented herein.

Dr. Andréa Diniz Lopes has no financial or proprietary interest in the materials presented herein.

Dr. Adam Lutz has no financial or proprietary interest in the materials presented herein.

Dr. Lee N. Marinko has no financial or proprietary interest in the materials presented herein.

Michael T. McKenney has no financial or proprietary interest in the materials presented herein.

Dr. Lori A. Michener has no financial or proprietary interest in the materials presented herein.

Dr. Joseph B. Myers has no financial or proprietary interest in the materials presented herein.

Dr. Thomas W. Nesser has no financial or proprietary interest in the materials presented herein.

Dr. Jonathan K. Park has no financial or proprietary interest in the materials presented herein.

Dr. Gail P. Parr has no financial or proprietary interest in the materials presented herein.

Dr. Brian J. Phillips has no financial or proprietary interest in the materials presented herein.

Kelsey Picha has no financial or proprietary interest in the materials presented herein.

Dr. Michael T. Piercey has no financial or proprietary interest in the materials presented herein.

Dr. Eric L. Sauers has no financial or proprietary interest in the materials presented herein.

Aaron Sciascia has no financial or proprietary interest in the materials presented herein.

Michael A. Shaffer has no financial or proprietary interest in the materials presented herein.

Dr. Ellen Shanley has no financial or proprietary interest in the materials presented herein.

Dr. Alison R. Snyder Valier has no financial or proprietary interest in the materials presented herein.

Dr. Angela Tate has no financial or proprietary interest in the materials presented herein.

Dr. Chuck Thigpen has no financial or proprietary interest in the materials presented herein.

Dr. W. Steven Tucker has no financial or proprietary interest in the materials presented herein.

Dr. Tim L. Uhl has no financial or proprietary interest in the materials presented herein.

Dr. Matthew K. Walsworth has no financial or proprietary interest in the materials presented herein.

INDEX